Advances in Oral Tissue Engineering

Advances in Oral Tissue Engineering

Edited by

Masaru Murata, DDS, PhD

Associate Professor and Senior Consultant of
Maxillofacial Implant Surgery
Division of Oral and Maxillofacial Surgery
Health Sciences University of Hokkaido
Tobetsu, Japan

Visiting Professor
Pioneer Dental College
Dhaka, Bangladesh

In-Woong Um, DDS, PhD

Director of Research and Development Institute
Korea Tooth Bank

Secretary General
Korea Auto-Tooth and Bone Bank
Seoul, Korea

quintessence books

Quintessence Publishing Co, Inc

Chicago, Berlin, Tokyo, London, Paris, Milan, Barcelona, Beijing, Istanbul, Moscow, New Delhi, Prague, São Paulo, Seoul, Singapore, and Warsaw

Library of Congress Cataloging-in-Publication Data

Advances in oral tissue engineering / edited by Masaru Murata and In-Woong Um.
p. ; cm.
Includes bibliographical references.
ISBN 978-0-86715-648-5 (softcover)
I. Murata, Masaru, editor. II. Um, In-Woong, editor.
[DNLM: 1. Dental Implants. 2. Tissue Engineering. 3. Bone Morphogenetic Protein Receptors. 4. Dental Implantation. WU 640]
RK667.I45
617.6'93--dc23

2014012525

Quintessence Publishing Co, Inc
4350 Chandler Drive
Hanover Park, IL 60133
www.quintpub.com

5 4 3 2 1

Editor: Bryn Grisham
Cover design: Ted Pereda
Production: Kaye Clemens

Printed in the USA

Contents

Foreword

Bone grafts have been employed for more than 100 years to restore discontinuity defects with bone loss such as traumatic defects, congenital deformities, and tumor resections, as well as for bone contouring, augmentation, or strengthening or as a scaffold. Today, research focuses more on using bone graft materials, growth factors, and stem cells to acquire a long-lasting bone volume and shape, especially in dental implant surgery.

For bone grafts used with simultaneous implant placement, it may take years to learn the feasibility of particular graft materials. Bone heals by vascularization, and the healing mechanism involves the process of adaptation and remodeling, which can affect the condition of grafted materials for several years with continued implant function and muscle use around the bony structures.

For many decades, researchers have tried to develop materials that could be used just like autogenous bone. Greater understanding of bone biology has made it possible to assemble experts in dentin research to produce this text and show that the basic biologic phenomena of dentin can be applied to bone grafts in implant dentistry to offer better clinical outcomes.

Pioneers in the field of dentin grafts are referred to in the text. The factors in dentin that cause induction of bone have been described for the past 40 years, and the persistent work in this area by Drs Masaru Murata and In-Woong Um has led to the successful purification of bone morphogenetic proteins in human dentin as we know it today. Consequently, continued studies in clinical application have produced promising outcomes. The future of our profession will experience a dramatic paradigm shift by using dentin and its derivatives as ideal graft materials.

Bone repair using dentin grafts, growth factors, stimulating factors, inductive factors, and other factors in clinical applications are all well described by authorities in the field. Some of these methods may seem far-fetched when considered in isolation. However, when the underlying concepts are considered together, clinical application of such materials in the clinical setting seems feasible. This book represents the first small step of dentin work and will lead to a great leap in dentistry around the world.

It is my sincere hope that this book will provide the profession with a scientifically based and clinically relevant resource for the emerging technique of autogenous tooth bone grafting.

Kyung-Wook Kim, DDS, MSD, PhD
Chair Commissioner
Korea Auto-Tooth and Bone Bank

Head and Professor
Department of Oral and Maxillofacial Surgery
College of Dentistry at Dankook University
Cheonan, Korea

Preface

Oral surgeons often consult with patients who have lost significant oral function and morphology and require bone surgery. Awareness of this predicament has guided our research for the last 25 years, and our team has focused on bone tissue regeneration induced by dentin and bone and resorbable bone substitutes.

The advanced topic of tissue regeneration commands worldwide attention, and the recent developments in regenerative bone surgery relating to biomaterials science are outstanding and dramatic. For example, the practice of "bio-recycling" natural tooth—a dental innovation of the 21st century—allows clinicians to reuse extracted teeth as intelligent biomaterials in bone regeneration. Natural teeth are an exceptional patient resource, and tooth-derived materials can contribute to successful bone regeneration while also allowing clinicians to feel good about reusing extracted teeth.

The research gathered in this book showcases excellent outcomes based on basic science and pioneering clinical application. New techniques using the tooth materials—especially dentin—provide realistic and practical regenerative treatments for all patients. I hope that this book will promote the concept of bio-recycling tooth in regenerative treatments and will serve as a stimulus for further study by ambitious researchers and clinicians.

In the immortal words of Kanzo Uchimura (1925), "dentistry is a work of love."

Acknowledgments

I would like to acknowledge the exceptional work and collaboration of all of the contributors to this book, the editorial help of Bryn Grisham at Quintessence Publishing, and my wife, Kyoko (1958–2013).

I must also thank Korea Tooth Bank for its support and the Japan Science and Technology Agency and Japan Ministry of Economy Trade and Industry for our grant. There are no borders in science.

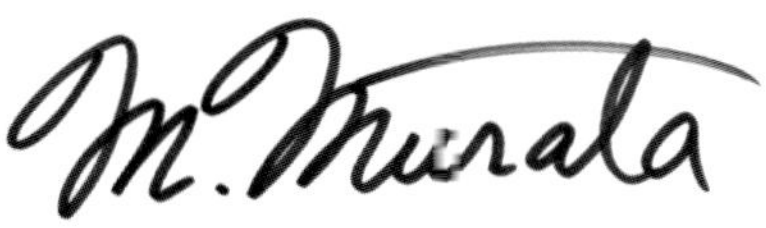

Masaru Murata, DDS, PhD

Contributors

Toshiyuki Akazawa, PhD
Senior Research Manager
Group of Polymer and Ceramics Materials
Industrial Research Institute
Hokkaido Research Organization
Sapporo, Japan

Toshiya Arakawa, PhD
Lecturer
Division of Oral Biochemistry
Health Sciences University of Hokkaido
Tobetsu, Japan

Makato Arisue, DDS, PhD
Professor and Senior Consultant of Oral and Maxillofacial Surgery
Division of Oral and Maxillofacial Surgery
Health Sciences University of Hokkaido
Tobetsu, Japan

Izumi Asahina, DDS, PhD
Professor and Chairman
Department of Regenerative Oral Surgery
Nagasaki University Graduate School of Biomedical Sciences
Nagasaki, Japan

Kazuhiko Endo, PhD
Professor and Chairman
Division of Biomaterials and Bioengineering
Health Sciences University of Hokkaido
Tobetsu, Japan

Mari Fujita, DDS, PhD
Assistant Professor
Division of Oral Microbiology
Health Sciences University of Hokkaido
Tobetsu, Japan

Youssef Haikel, DDS, PhD
Professor
INSERM U977 and Department of Operative Dentistry and Endodontics
University of Strasbourg
Strasbourg, France

Shingo Hara, DDS, PhD
Medical Director
Department of Dentistry and Oral and Maxillofacial Surgery
Kochi Health Sciences Center
Kochi, Japan

Jun Hino, DDS, PhD
Assistant Professor
Division of Reconstructive Surgery for Oral and Maxillofacial Region
Health Sciences University of Hokkaido
Tobetsu, Japan

Akira Ishisaki, DDS, PhD
Professor
Department of Biochemistry
Division of Cellular Biosignal Sciences
Iwate Medical University
Morioka, Japan

Katsutoshi Ito, DDS, PhD
Assistant Professor
Division of Oral and Maxillofacial Surgery
Health Sciences University of Hokkaido
Tobetsu, Japan

Md Arafat Kabir, DDS
Doctoral Student
Division of Oral and Maxillofacial Surgery
Health Sciences University of Hokkaido
Tobetsu, Japan

Yoji Kamiura, DDS, PhD
Private Practice
Otaru, Japan

Clinical Professor
Hokkaido University
Sapporo, Japan

Masamitsu Kawanami, DDS, PhD
Professor
Department of Periodontology and Endodontology
Hokkaido University Graduate School of Dental Medicine
Sapporo, Japan

Masahiko Kikuchi
General Manager
Mutoh Company
Tokyo, Japan

Kyung-Wook Kim, DDS, MSD, PhD
Chair Commissioner
Korea Auto-Tooth and Bone Bank

Head and Professor
Department of Oral and Maxillofacial Surgery
College of Dentistry at Dankook University
Cheonan, Korea

Myung-Jin Kim, DDS, MSD, PhD
Professor
Department of Oral and Maxillofacial Surgery
Seoul National University School of Dentistry
Seoul, Korea

Young-Kyun Kim, DDS, PhD
Professor of Oral and Maxillofacial Surgery
Section of Dentistry
Seoul National University Bundang Hospital
Seongnam, Korea

Morihiro Kimura, DDS PhD
Private Practice in Periodontics
Chiba, Japan

Clinical Professor
Health Sciences University of Hokkaido
Tobetsu, Japan

Ryuichiro Kumazawa, DDS PhD
Private Practice in Oral and Maxillofacial Surgery
Otaru, Japan

Takaki Kumazawa, DDS, PhD
Private Practice
Otaru, Japan

Kaoru Kusano, DDS, PhD
Lecturer
Division of Oral and Maxillofacial Surgery
Health Sciences University of Hokkaido
Tobetsu, Japan

Jingo Kusukawa, DDS, PhD
Professor and Senior Consultant of Oral and Maxillofacial Surgery
Dental and Oral Medical Centre
Kurume University School of Medicine
Kurume, Japan

Bu-Kyu Lee, DDS, MS, PhD
Associate Professor
Department of Oral and Maxillofacial Surgery
Asan Medical Center
University of Ulsan College of Medicine
Seoul, Korea

Jeong-Keun Lee, DDS, PhD
Professor
Division of Oral and Maxillofacial Surgery
Ajou University School of Medicine

Vice Dean of Academic Affairs
Ajou University Graduate School of Clinical Dentistry
Suwon, Korea

Hervé Lesot, PhD
Associate Professor
INSERM U424
University of Strasbourg
Strasbourg, France

Yasuhito Minamida, DDS
Doctoral Student
Division of Oral and Maxillofacial Surgery
Health Sciences University of Hokkaido
Tobetsu, Japan

Masaharu Mitsugi, DDS, PhD
Advisor and Oral and Maxillofacial Surgeon
Takamatsu Oral and Maxillofacial Clinic
Kochi Health Sciences Center, Kure Kyosai Hospital

Secretary General
Japan Auto-Tooth and Bone Bank
Kochi, Japan

Visiting Professor
Laos National University
Vientiane, Laos

Hirofumi Miyaji, DDS, PhD
Lecturer
Department of Periodontology and Endodontology
Hokkaido University Graduate School of Dental Medicine
Sapporo, Japan

Hiroshi Miyakawa, PhD
Associate Professor
Division of Oral Microbiology
Health Sciences University of Hokkaido
Tobetsu, Japan

Masaru Murata, DDS, PhD
Associate Professor and Senior Consultant of Maxillofacial Implant Surgery
Division of Oral and Maxillofacial Surgery
Health Sciences University of Hokkaido
Tobetsu, Japan

Visiting Professor
Pioneer Dental College
Dhaka, Bangladesh

Noriyuki Nagai, DDS, PhD
Professor Emeritus
Division of Oral Pathology
Okayama University
Okayama, Japan

Futami Nagano-Takebe, DDS, PhD
Assistant Professor
Division of Biomaterials and Bioengineering
Health Sciences University of Hokkaido
Tobetsu, Japan

Sumiyoshi Naito
Chief Medical Technologist
Clinical Laboratory
Dental and Internal Medical Clinic
Health Sciences University of Hokkaido
Tobetsu, Japan

Katsuo Nakamura
Senior Staff
Industrial Research Institute
Hokkaido Research Organization
Sapporo, Japan

Futoshi Nakazawa, PhD
Professor
Division of Oral Microbiology
Health Sciences University of Hokkaido
Tobetsu, Japan

Naoto Okubo, DDS, PhD
Postdoctoral Fellow
Department of Pathophysiology and Therapeutics
Division of Pharmasciences
Hokkaido University
Sapporo, Japan

Jean-Victor Ruch, MD, PhD (1935–2003)
Professor of Embryology
Director of the Institute of Medical Biology
Faculty of Medicine
University of Louis Pasteur
Strasbourg, France

Denis Selimovic, MD, PhD
Associate Professor
Department of Operative Dentistry and Endodontics
University of Strasbourg
Strasbourg, France

Takanori Shibata, DDS, PhD
Professor and Senior Consultant of Oral and Maxillofacial Surgery
Division of Reconstructive Surgery for Oral and Maxillofacial Region
Health Sciences University of Hokkaido
Tobetsu, Japan

Taishin Takuma, PhD
Professor
Division of Oral Biochemistry
Health Sciences University of Hokkaido
Tobetsu, Japan

Junichi Tazaki, DDS, PhD
Assistant Professor
Division of Reconstructive Surgery for Oral and Maxillofacial Region
Health Sciences University of Hokkaido
Tobetsu, Japan

Hidetsugu Tsujigiwa, PhD
Associate Professor
Division of Oral Pathology
Okayama University
Okayama, Japan

Osamu Uehara, DDS, PhD
Assistant Professor
Division of Disease Control and Molecular Epidemioloy
Health Sciences University of Hokkaido
Tobetsu, Japan

In-Woong Um, DDS, PhD
Director of Research and Development Institute
Korea Tooth Bank

Secretary General
Korea Auto-Tooth and Bone Bank
Seoul, Korea

1

Bone Autografting

Jingo Kusukawa

The augmentation of alveolar ridges is now considered a predictable procedure, with a variety of grafting materials available for the surgeon to use. Among them, autologous bone grafting is the gold standard for bone augmentation. The patient's own living bone has desirable properties, including osteoinduction, osteoconduction, and osteogenesis. The only disadvantages of autologous grafting are donor site injury and the limited amounts of bone available for harvest without excessive donor site morbidity. The donor site for grafted bone should be chosen according to the type of bony defect. In addition to hard tissue management, soft tissue management at the bone graft site is also important for successful bone augmentation.

Histology of Bone

Bone consists of both organic and inorganic substances (Figs 1-1 and 1-2). The organic part of bone constitutes approximately 30% of bone. The organic matrix of bone comprises 90% type I collagen, and the remaining 10% is noncollagenous proteins, such as osteonectin, osteopontin, and proteoglycans. Sixty-five percent to 70% of bone is made up of inorganic substances, primarily hydroxyapatite ($Ca_{10}[PO_4]_6[OH]_2$).

Bone can be classified as *cortical* or *cancellous*. Cortical bone is the hard outer layer of bone, which is dense and compact and contains a series of haversian systems (osteons), with lacunae housing osteocytes. The outer surface of the cortical bone is covered with periosteum, which contains osteoblasts and progenitor cells in its inner surface or cambium layer. The periosteum provides the blood supply via Volkmann canals that are connected to the haversian system. Filling the interior of the bone is the cancellous bone (also known as *trabecular bone* or *spongy bone*), which consists of a network of trabeculae and fills the marrow space between the cortices. Cancellous bone houses the cells that are responsible for bone turnover and regeneration. The lining of the internal surface of the bone, the *endosteum*, also contains osteoblasts and osteoprogenitor cells. Bone marrow contains not only hematopoietic tissue but also blood vessels and stromal tissue, including fibroblasts, adipocytes, osteoblasts, osteoclasts, and mesenchymal progenitor cells. During aging, bone marrow reduces the number of progenitor cells of hematopoietic and stromal tissue and is substituted by fat.

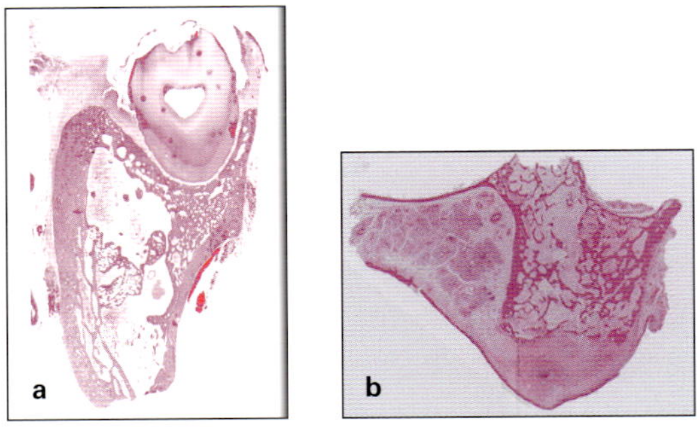

Fig 1-1 Cross section of mandibular bone *(a)* and maxillary bone *(b)*.

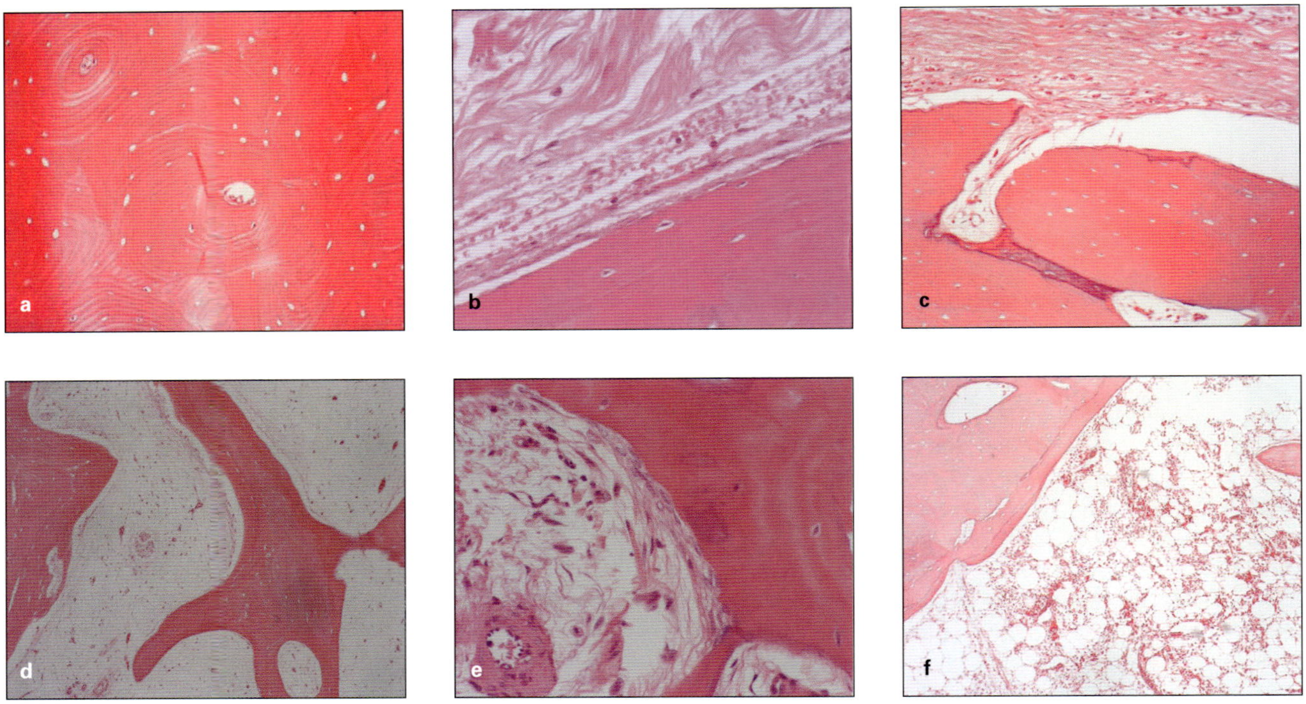

Fig 1-2 Histology of jawbone. *(a)* Cortical bone consisting of haversian systems (osteon) with lacunae housing osteocytes that concentrically line the haversian canal (hematoxylin-eosin [HE]; ×40). *(b)* The periosteum covering the outer surface of the cortical bone consists of two layers. The inner layer (cambium) contains osteoblasts and progenitor cells (HE; ×200). *(c)* The periosteum provides the blood supply through Volkmann canals connected to the haversian system (HE; ×40). *(d)* Cancellous bone tissue (trabecular bone, spongy bone) consists of a network of trabeculae that fills the marrow (HE; ×40). *(e)* Endosteum, lining the internal surface of the cancellous bone, contains osteoblasts and osteoprogenitor cells (HE; ×200). *(f)* Bone marrow contains hematopoietic tissue, blood vessels, and stromal tissue (HE; ×40).

Healing of Grafted Bone

Bone healing can be classified into *primary* and *secondary healing*. Primary bone healing implies direct contact or a gap less than 1 mm between bone fragments. Following removal of bone by osteoclasts at the front of the cutting cone, osteoblasts secrete osteoid and lay down new bone. Secondary healing of bone can be divided into three stages. In the early inflammatory stage, there is formation of a hematoma between bone fragments. Inflammatory cells and fibroblasts invade the hematoma, which eventually becomes granulation tissue. Second, revascularization and ingrowth of bone-promoting cells in the granulation tissue occur. Osteoinductive substances bring these osteogenic cells into the space, and an osteoconductive material filling the space works as a scaffold for these cells. The osteoblasts lay down osteoid and form the callus, which eventually ossifies. Finally, remodeling of bone occurs over months to years.

Cortical bone features superior structural strength but has fewer osteoblasts and osteocytes and less surface area per unit weight, and it serves as a barrier to vascular ingrowth and remodeling compared with cancellous bone. Cortical bone grafts heal by a process of "creeping substitution" that is similar to primary bone healing. After a nonvascularized cortical bone graft is transferred to a defect, the grafted material is

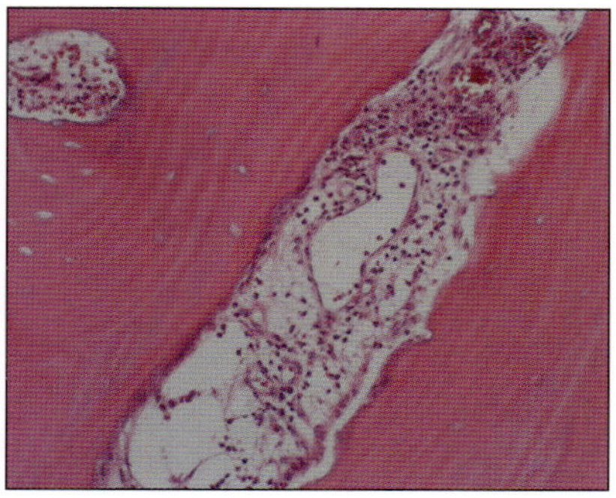

Fig 1-3 Necrotic center of a cortical bone graft. The grafted cortical bone has lost osteocytes in the lacunae, and osteoblastic cells, vessels, and inflammatory cells in the graft bone are observed (HE; ×100).

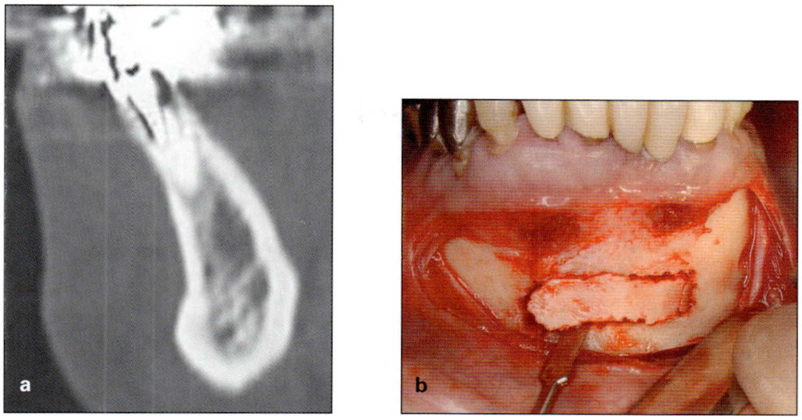

Fig 1-4 *(a)* Cross-sectional computed tomographic view of the mandibular symphyseal region. Monocortical and cancellous bone blocks can be harvested from the mandibular symphysis. *(b)* An osteotomy of the labial cortical bone can be made with a small round fissure bur, electric surgical saw, or piezoelectric surgical device.

slowly resorbed by osteoclasts and simultaneously replaced with new bone created by osteoblasts. This process of bone apposition and remodeling eventually results in the replacement of the grafted material; however, the grafted bone remains at the necrotic center (Fig 1-3) mixed with the newly formed bone. The majority of osteocytes in cortical bone do not survive grafting, and neovascularization of nonvital grafted bone is difficult.[1]

In particulate cancellous bone grafts, the grafted material provides an adequate scaffold for ingrowth of osteoblasts and vascular cells and for the apposition of bone, and revascularization proceeds faster than in cortical bone grafts. Thus, a particulate cancellous bone and marrow graft shows fast bone regeneration, resistance to infection, and ease in handling.

Bone grafts are also strongly influenced by mechanical forces during the remodeling stage.[2] To prevent excessive resorption of a graft and allow for new bone formation, clinicians should contain or fix the material at the site according to the type of defect and graft material used. To promote good healing of a wound, the grafted bone must be contained by healthy bone and periosteum.

Bone Grafting

Type of bone defect

The type of bone defect strongly influences the grafting material and technique that will be used for reconstruction. Bone defects are simply divided into horizontal and vertical types according to the direction of alveolar bone loss. Vertical bone loss is more complicated to reconstruct than horizontal bone loss. The number of bony walls remaining at the site to be grafted is relevant to the difficulty of grafting.

Graft donor sites

When selecting the source of a bone graft, the surgeon must consider multiple factors with regard to the recipient site, the donor site, and the patient. The donor site should be chosen on the basis of quantity, quality, and form of the bone required. The size of the defect to be restored is a major factor in determining the quantity of grafting material required. The type of defect is also relevant to the quality of graft required, ie, cortical or cancellous. Donor site morbidity is an important factor to be considered for the patient. Some extraoral donor sites, such as the anterior iliac crest or the tibia, enable two surgical teams to work simultaneously at the recipient site and the donor site; in contrast, harvesting from the posterior iliac crest requires that the patient be repositioned during surgery, prior to grafting to an intraoral site. The volume of bone available for harvesting varies depending on the donor site.

Intraoral bone harvesting has the advantage of being carried out in the same operative field under local anesthesia; however, the quantity of material that can be harvested is limited. To make up for deficient volumes of graft bone, combination with allograft, xenograft, or synthetic graft is a useful option.

Mandibular symphysis

The mandibular symphysis is one of the most commonly used sources of bone graft (Fig 1-4). There are two incision designs to approach the symphysis: sulcular and vestibular. Care must be taken to avoid injury to the mental nerve and teeth. The vestibular incision is associated with wound dehiscence, scar formation, persistent postoperative discomfort of the wound, and possible chin ptosis, whereas the sulcular incision might contribute to gingival recession.

A monocortical labial osteotomy in the mandibular symphysis is performed from 5 mm anterior to the mental fora-

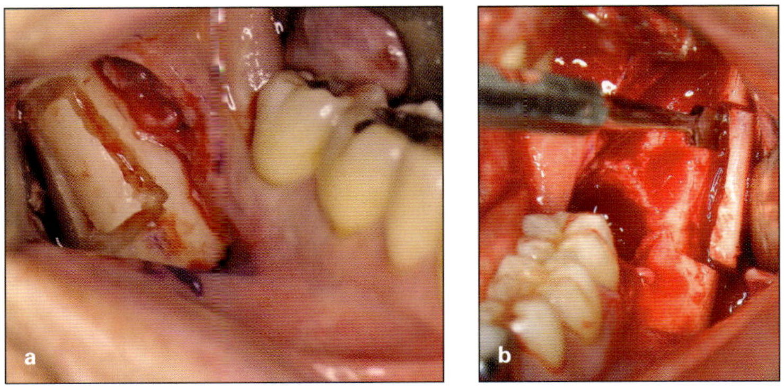

Fig 1-5 The ascending mandibular ramus and body are useful sources of donor bone. *(a)* A mucosal incision was made along the anterior border of the ramus, and the outer cortical layer was harvested. *(b)* Cortical bone harvesting from the posterior mandibular body and third molar extraction were performed simultaneously.

men to the midline, anterior to the inferior border of the mandible, and superiorly at least 5 mm below the root apices of the anterior teeth, on each side of the mental region. A corticocancellous bone block can be harvested. A quantitative anatomical study revealed that the average block size was 20.9 × 9.9 × 6.9 mm; the smallest block was 21.0 × 6.5 × 6.0 mm, and the largest was 25.0 × 13.0 × 9.0 mm.[3]

Mandibular ramus and body

The region from the anterior border of the ramus to the posterior part of the mandibular body is a sufficient source of compact bone (Fig 1-5). The incision for an approach to the mandibular ramus is begun at the alveolar mucosa of the posterior molar and extended posteriorly, to the ascending ramus. Following a releasing incision of the buccinator muscle at the anterior border of the ascending ramus, the temporalis muscle is stripped off to prevent herniation of the buccal fat pad. After the lateral wall of the mandibular ramus has been exposed, the osteotomy lines should be marked by a surgical pen or fissure bur. Osteotomies of the lateral cortical bone are then made at the middle of the ramus superiorly and at the first or second molar region inferiorly. The width of bone to be harvested should be no more than one-third of the width of the mandibular ramus. Each groove is then connected at the depth of the lateral cortical bone medial to the external oblique ridge. Harvesting is completed with a careful split from the donor site by means of a small flat chisel; this prevents injury to the infra-alveolar nerves and vessels.

Zygomatic buttress

Bone blocks harvested from the zygomatic buttress are of good quality, but quantity is reduced and therefore suitable only for one- or two-tooth edentulous sites. Easy access is offered with a vestibular incision from the canine to the first molar. A bone block of 1 cm^3 can be harvested at the base of the zygomaticoalveolar crest. Attention should be paid to prevent injury to the maxillary sinus membrane at the time of bone harvest.

Maxillary tuberosity and retromolar pad

Cancellous bone can be harvested easily from the maxillary tuberosity and retromolar pads with bone forceps or an osteotrite, but the quantity obtained is small. Gentle handling must be done to prevent perforation of the lingual aspect of the mandible.

Tori (exostosis)

The torus palatinus, torus mandibularis, and alveolar tori are available as sources of bone grafting (Fig 1-6). Because the bone in the exostosis is hard and compact, any excised bone specimens should be crushed with a bone mill before use as graft material.

Others

Bone blocks can be harvested from the inferior border of the mandible (Fig 1-7) and the coronoid process.

Grafting techniques

To allow for new bone formation, a graft must be contained at the defect site and in contact with healthy surrounding tissue. When attempting vertical augmentation, it is more difficult to contain graft materials at the site and to maintain the shape and space of the alveolus for bone formation.

Socket grafting

A fresh extraction socket, which has five walls of native bone, provides superior containment of particulate bone graft material. The socket should be cleaned with a dental curette before grafting and then filled with graft materials as densely as possible. To prevent infection, the wound should be closed with a mucoperiosteal flap, with or without a resorbable membrane such as collagen, to prevent exposure to the oral environment (Fig 1-8).

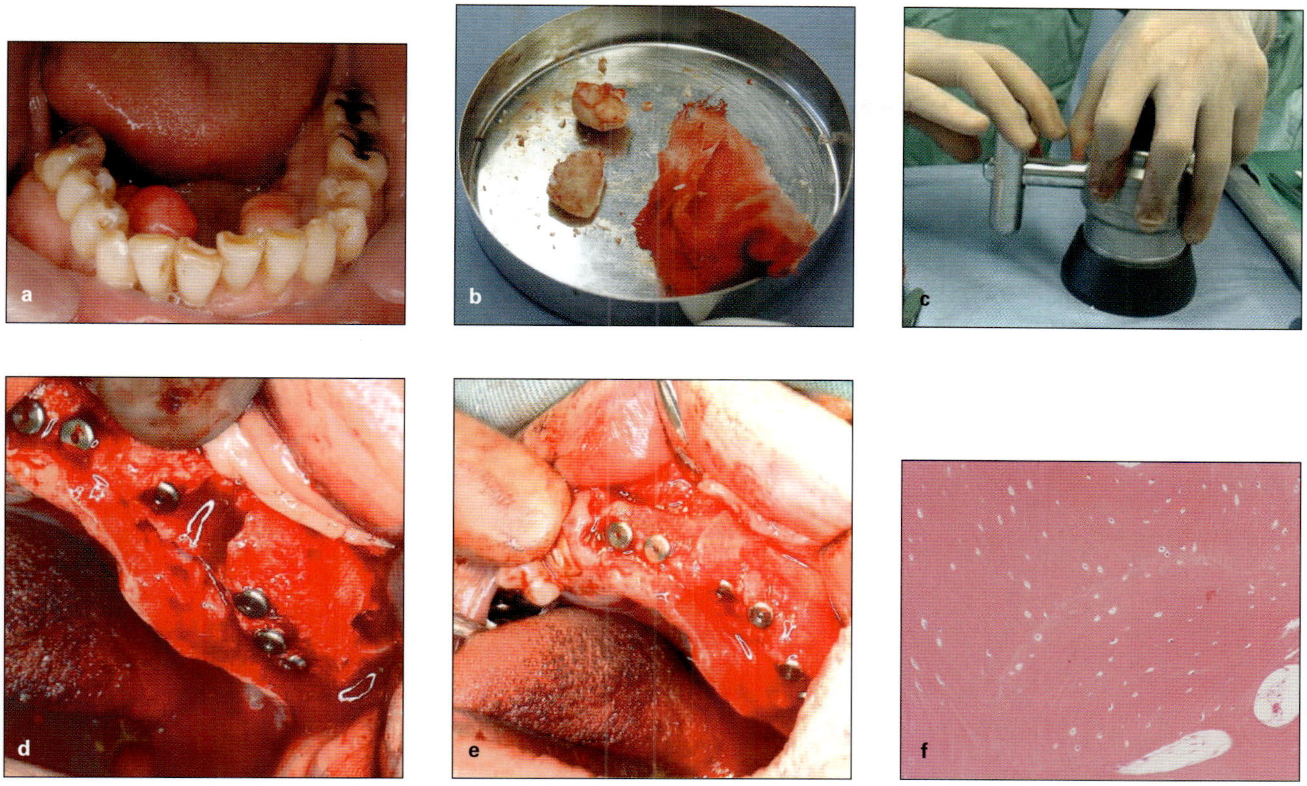

Fig 1-6 *(a to c)* The mandibular tori were excised and crushed with a bone mill. *(d,e)* The bone graft obtained was packed into the defect created after tooth extraction. *(f)* Histologic view of the mandibular tori shows compact bone (HE; × 40).

Fig 1-7 *(a,b)* A bone block was harvested from the inferior border of the mandible for grafting in the atrophic maxillary alveolus. *(c)* A curved cortical bone block that matched the curve of the alveolus was obtained. *(d,e)* The bone graft was fixed to the basal bone with a miniplate and implants.

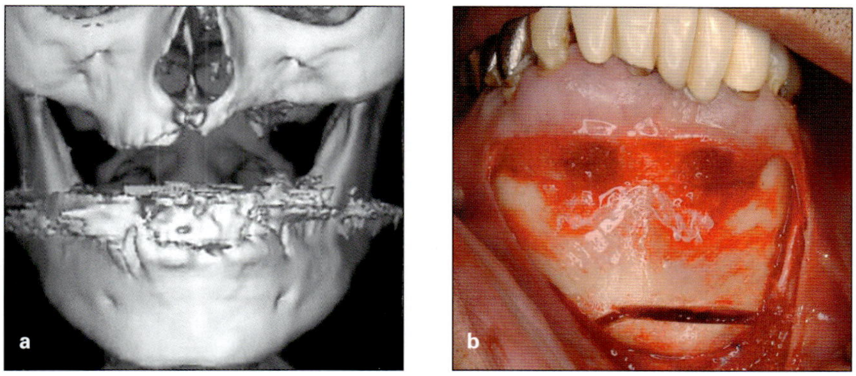

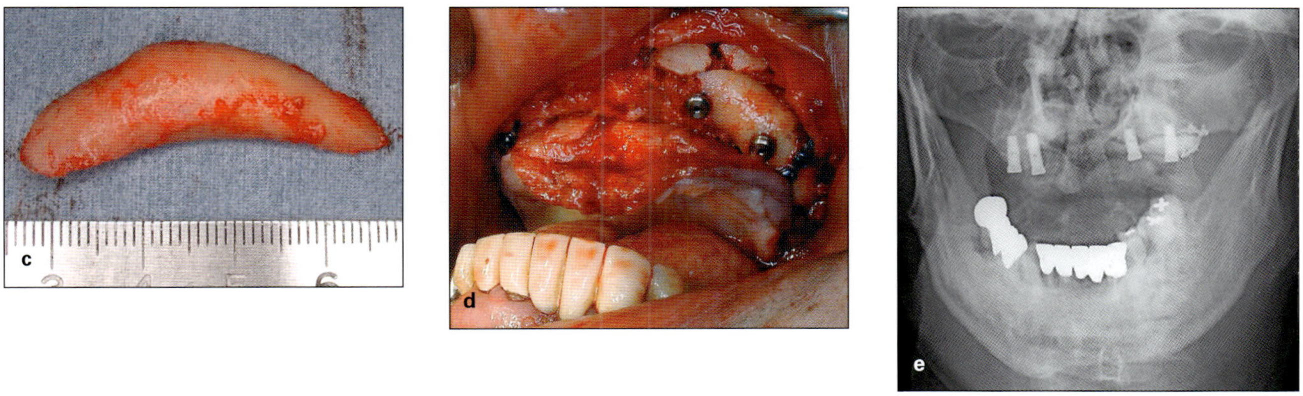

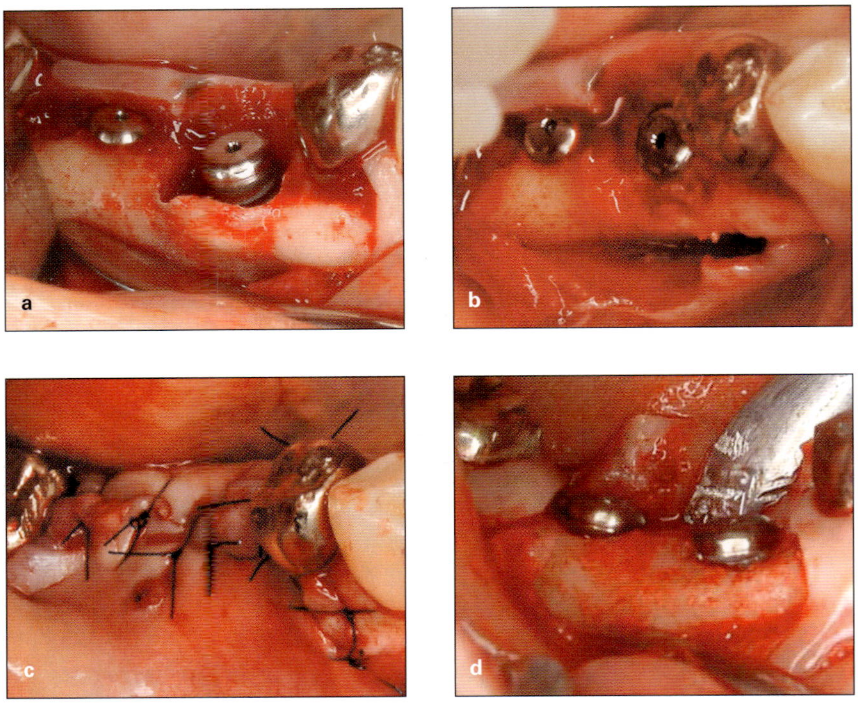

Fig 1-8 *(a)* Socket grafting with immediate implant placement. *(b)* Particulate bone was packed into the space between the extraction socket and the implant body, and *(c)* the wound was covered completely with a mucoperiosteal flap. *(d)* Sufficient bone had formed around the implant 4 months after grafting.

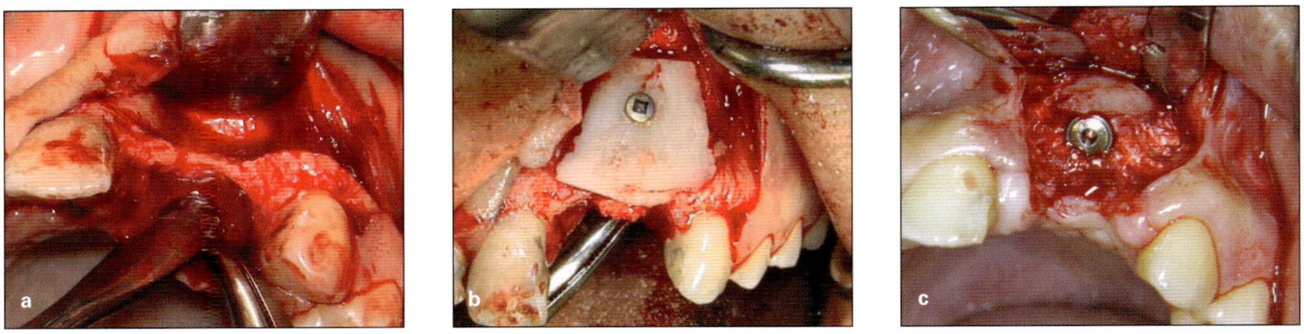

Fig 1-9 *(a,b)* After trauma, the loss of alveolar bone was augmented by veneer grafting with cortical bone. *(c)* Although the site at 6 months postoperative demonstrated partial resorption at the edge of the graft bone, an implant was successfully placed at the site, with additional hydroxyapatite particulate graft used to fill the area.

Horizontal ridge augmentation by veneer bone grafting

Veneer grafting is a popular method for the repair of atrophied anterior maxillae (Fig 1-9). A simple method to increase the width of the alveolus is to place a cortical block, which can be fixed directly to the host bone with microscrews. In screw insertion, care should be taken to avoid injury to the dental roots. Any remaining gap between the graft and the host bone can be filled with particulate graft.

Vertical ridge augmentation by onlay bone grafting

Vertically and horizontally deficient ridges can be restored with onlay block corticocancellous grafts. The most suitable donor site for full-arch onlay grafts is the iliac crest (Fig 1-10). To ensure graft survival, it is important to cover the bone graft with an intact periosteum. The mucoperiosteal flap should be designed to adequately expose the ridge to be augmented and to maintain sufficient vascular supply for the graft. A crestal or vestibular incision can be used to expose the ridge. Soft tissue management for tension-free primary closure is also important for graft survival.

Ridge augmentation with titanium mesh

The use of titanium mesh for osseous restoration of the atrophic alveolus was introduced by Boyne et al in 1985.[4] Titanium mesh has the advantages of morphologic flexibility and biologic affinity, and it acts as a barrier and provides physical support to the soft tissue over the bone graft. The

Fig 1-10 *(a)* A severe alveolar bone defect was created after excision of odontogenic myxoma of the mandible. *(b)* A corticocancellous bone block harvested from the anterior iliac crest was placed on the residual mandibular bone and fixed with the circumferential wiring technique. *(c)* To cover the augmented area, a split mucoperiosteal flap was created via a vestibular incision. *(d)* Postoperative view.

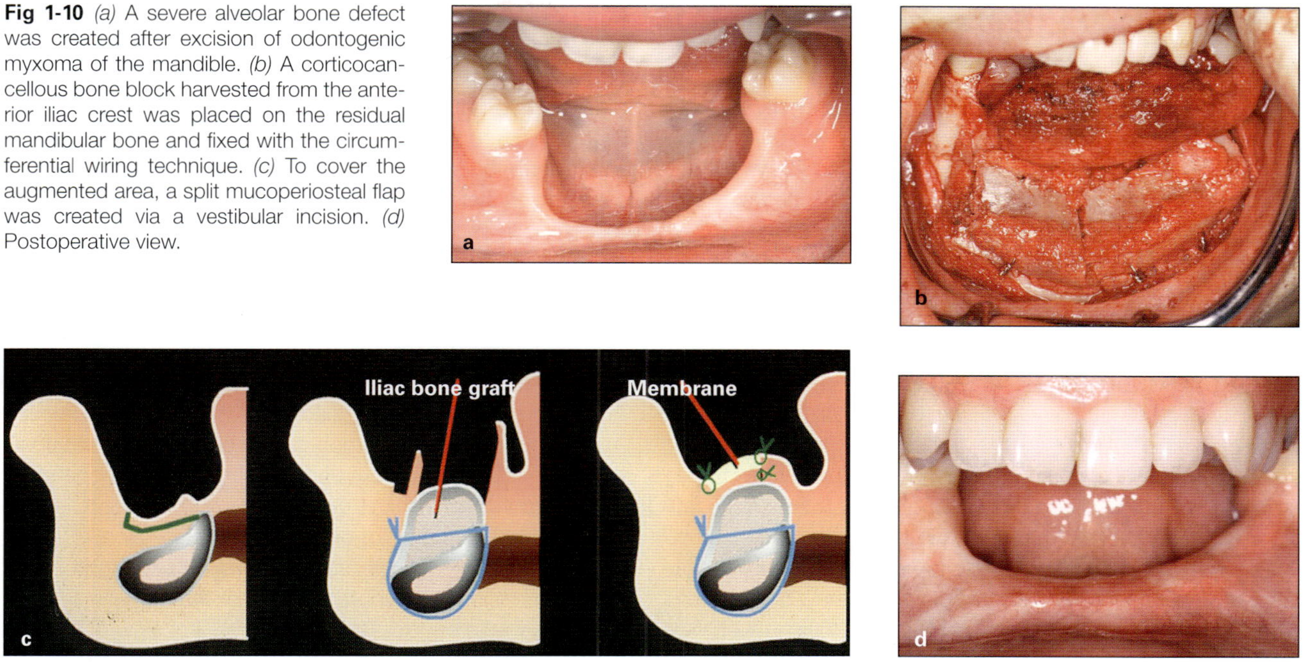

Fig 1-11 Augmentation of the atrophic edentulous maxilla by titanium mesh and particulate bone graft mixed with hydroxyapatite. *(a,b)* Cross-sectional computed tomographic images before and after surgery. *(c)* Titanium mesh and particulate bone graft in place on the right side of the upper alveolus. *(d)* Reconstructed maxillary ridge 6 months after bone grafting.

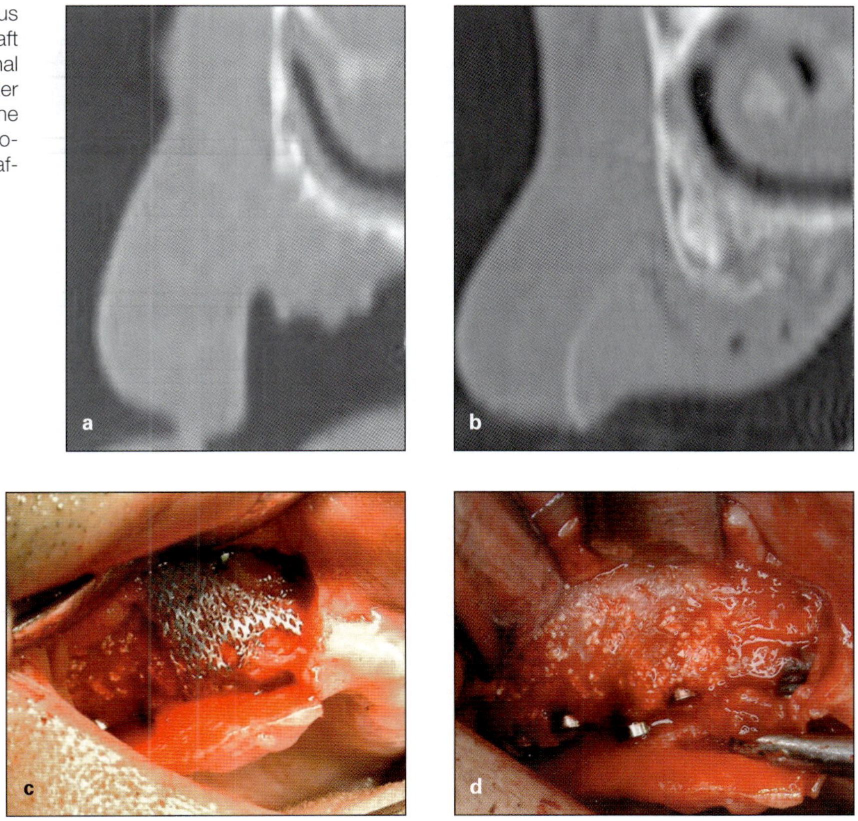

titanium mesh technique can be used for various types of graft materials, including autografts, allografts, xenografts, and alloplasts. Various types of titanium mesh are commercially available. The mesh is contoured and trimmed to eliminate any sharp areas that may injure nerves or overlying tissues. After the mesh tray has been packed densely with particulate grafting material, it is placed into position and fixed with microscrews (Figs 1-11 and 1-12). Even when there is exposure to the oral cavity, it rarely leads to total graft loss.[5]

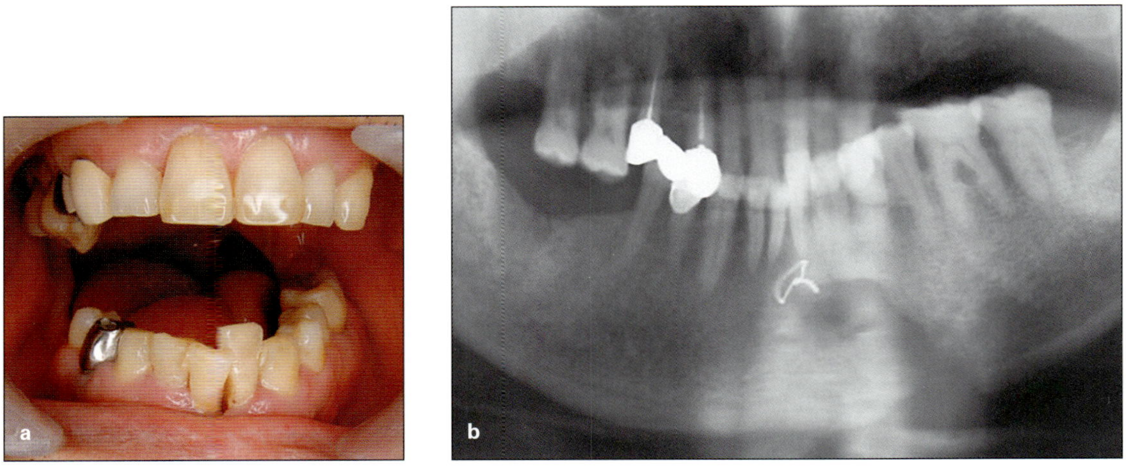

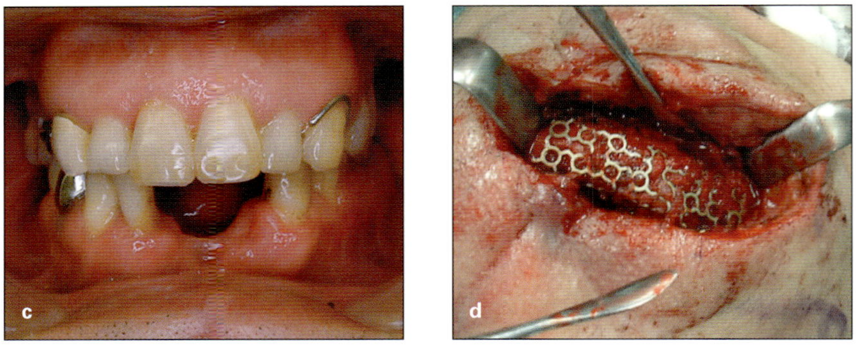

Fig 1-12 *(a,b)* Segmental bone loss of the mandible occurred after surgery for pharyngeal cancer. *(c to e)* After repositioning of the occlusion, the segmental defect was reconstructed with titanium mesh and particulate bone graft. *(f)* Mature bone had been created by 6 months after reconstructive surgery.

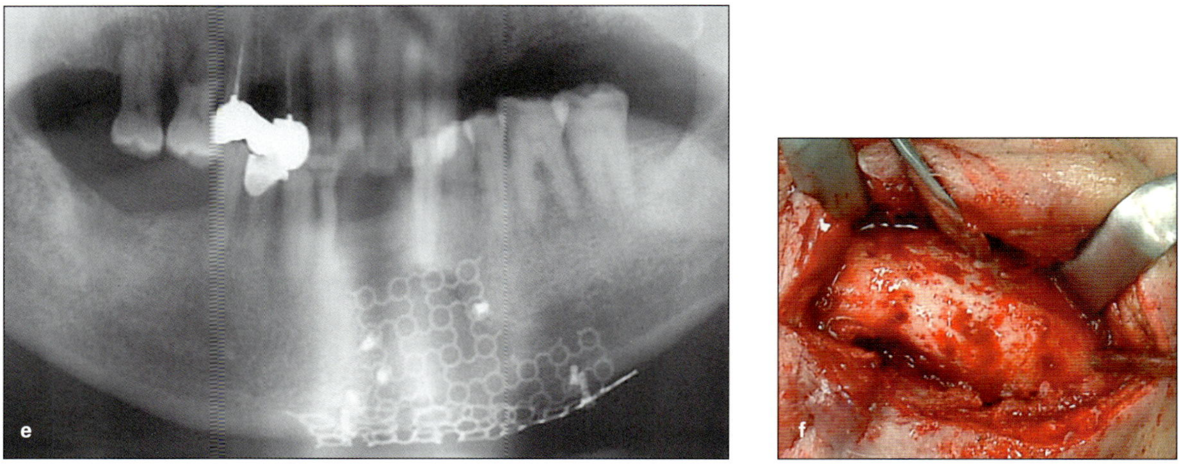

References

1. Acocella A, Bertolai R, Colafranceschi M, Sacco R. Clinical, histological and histomorphometric evaluation of the healing of mandibular ramus bone block grafts for alveolar ridge augmentation before implant placement. J Craniomaxillofac Surg 2010;38:222–230.
2. Wolff J. The Law of Bone Remodelling. Berlin: Springer-Verlag, 1986.
3. Montazem A, Valauri DV, St-Hilaire H, Buchbinder D. The mandibular symphysis as a donor site in maxillofacial bone grafting: A quantitative anatomic study. J Oral Maxillofac Surg 2000;58:1368–1371.
4. Boyne PJ, Cole MD, Stringer D, Shafqat JP. A technique for osseous restoration of deficient edentulous maxillary ridges. J Oral Maxillofac Surg 1985;43:87–91.
5. Louis PJ, Gutta R, Said-Al-Naief N, Bartolucci AA. Reconstruction of the maxilla and mandible with particulate bone graft and titanium mesh for implant placement. J Oral Maxillofac Surg 2008;66:235–245.

2

Angiogenic Capacity of Periodontal Ligament–Derived Stem Cells

Naoto Okubo, Akira Ishisaki

The periodontal ligament (PDL) is a specialized connective tissue that is located between the tooth root and alveolar bone. PDL tissue originates from neural crest–derived ectomesenchyme[1,2] and contains a heterogenous mixture of cell types, including PDL fibroblasts, cementoblasts, osteoblasts, epithelial cells (rests of Malassez), vascular endothelial cells (ECs), smooth muscle cells (SMCs), and certain types of nerve cells.[3] The PDL plays an important role in supporting tooth function: maintaining homeostasis. In response to oral pathologic and physiologic environmental alterations, such as periodontitis, trauma, and tooth movement by orthodontic treatment, PDL cells have the capacity to reconstruct the periodontal structure.

As a clinical example, a case for periodontal tissue reconstruction through the technique for guided tissue regeneration is shown in Fig 2-1. For the treatment of a three-wall intrabony defect that included the root apex and furcation, flap surgery was performed with guided tissue regeneration. A nonresorbable expanded polytetrafluoroethylene membrane was sutured over the intrabony defect to prevent the migration of undesired cells from the overlying soft tissues into the wound and to maintain the space for the desired bone regeneration without using any bone materials or platelet-rich plasma. Thirteen months after the membrane was removed, newly regenerated osseous tissue was seen to have filled the dead space of the defect area. This incredible process to regenerate a defect is brought about by the progenitor/stem cells derived in the remaining PDL tissue. With regard to scientific evidence, enamel matrix derivative, which is often used in periodontal surgery, has been reported to promote the activation of progenitor/stem cells in reconstructing PDL tissue.[4–7]

For a tissue to have reconstructive ability, multipotent progenitor cells or putative stem cells must be present. The paravascular zones in adult PDL contain the progenitors of fibroblastic and mineralized tissue–forming cell lineages, ie, the osteoblastic and cementoblastic lineages.[8] Recently, several studies have indicated that PDL fibroblastic cells have biologic characteristics in common with bone marrow mesenchymal cells, suggesting that the mineralized tissue lineages may have originated from a common early progenitor cell.[9–12] PDL cells have also shown cementoblastic/osteoblastic and adipogenic differentiation in vitro and have the potential to generate cementum/PDL-like tissue in vivo, suggesting that multipotent stem cells are present.[13] In contrast, it has been shown that bone marrow mesenchymal cells can give rise to both osteoblasts and SMCs.[14] Thus, it seems reasonable to suppose that both osteoblasts and SMCs may develop from the same progenitor and that multipotent stem cells in the PDL may differentiate not only into cementoblasts/osteoblasts but also into SMCs.

A blood supply is indispensable for the regeneration of damaged or lost PDL tissue.[15] Therefore, an understanding of how PDL tissue recruits the precursors of vascular cells and how the precursors then differentiate into vascular cells is necessary to establish a practical strategy to regenerate the damaged or lost PDL. With respect to blood vessels, their inner walls are constructed from two types of cells, ECs and SMCs. Recently, it was found

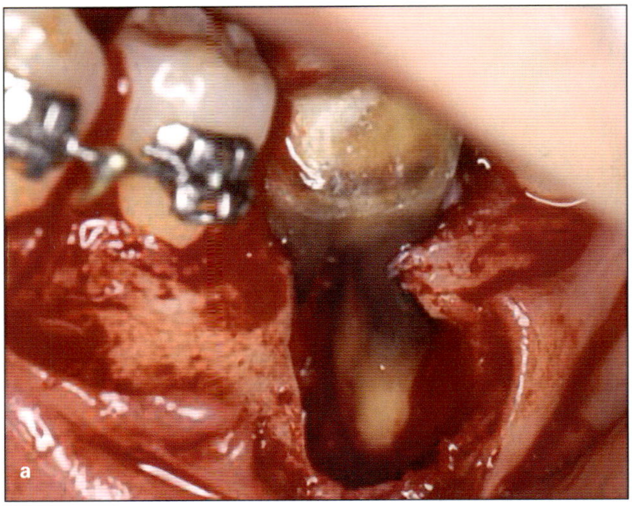

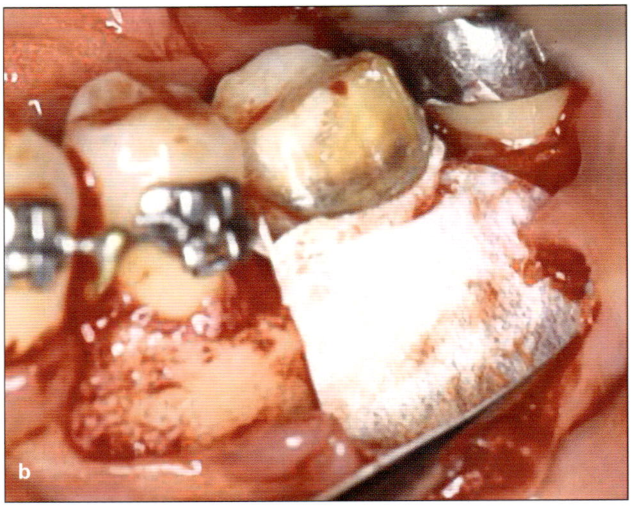

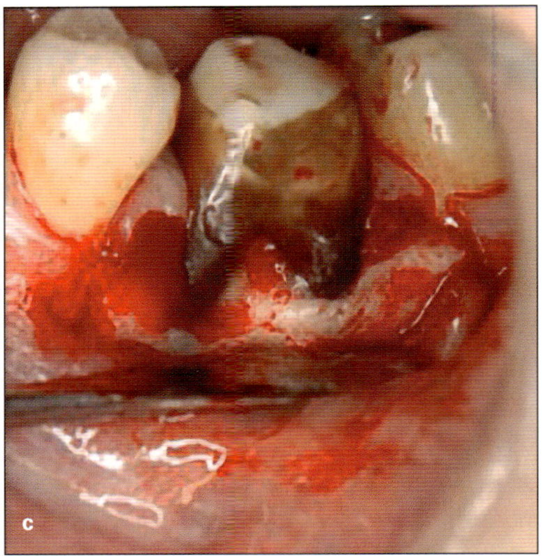

Fig 2-1 Guided tissue regeneration treatment of an alveolar bone defect. *(a)* The infected granulation tissue was removed, and curettage of the root surfaces was performed in an intrabony defect around the mandibular first molar. *(b)* After debridement of the infected tissue, a nonresorbable membrane was used to cover the intrabony defect. *(c)* Thirteen months after the membrane was removed, the intrabony defect was filled with regenerated osseous tissue. (Courtesy of Prof Kitetsu Shin, Saitama, Japan.)

that multipotent Flk-1–positive embryonic stem cells, pulmonary valve progenitor cells, and "side population" progenitor cells from arteries give rise to ECs and SMCs.[16] In addition, transdifferentiation of ECs to SMCs and of SMCs to ECs has been reported recently.[17,18] Thus, both ECs and SMCs develop from the same progenitor. These general observations on the progenitors of osteoblasts, ECs, and SMCs have led to the hypothesis that multipotent cells in the PDL may give rise to a vascular cell lineage rather than only osteoblastic/cementoblastic cell lineages.

However, it must be clarified whether the multipotent cells in the PDL have the ability to build the capillary network of blood vessels. The current chapter introduces the reader to new knowledge about the cells derived from PDL and their ability to construct blood vessel structures in a three-dimensional type I collagen scaffold.

Establishment and Characterization of Single Cell–Derived Cultures from Rat Fibroblasts Derived from PDL

The authors first established a primary culture of rat PDL fibroblasts. Then two types of single cell–derived cultures (SCDCs; SCDC1 and SCDC2) were obtained from the primary culture. As shown in Fig 2-2, primary rat PDL fibroblast (Fig 2-2a) and SCDCs (Figs 2-2b and 2-2c) have a fibroblastic spindle shape. The expression of markers for mesenchymal stem cells (MSCs), vascular ECs, and SMCs in each SCDC was investigated.

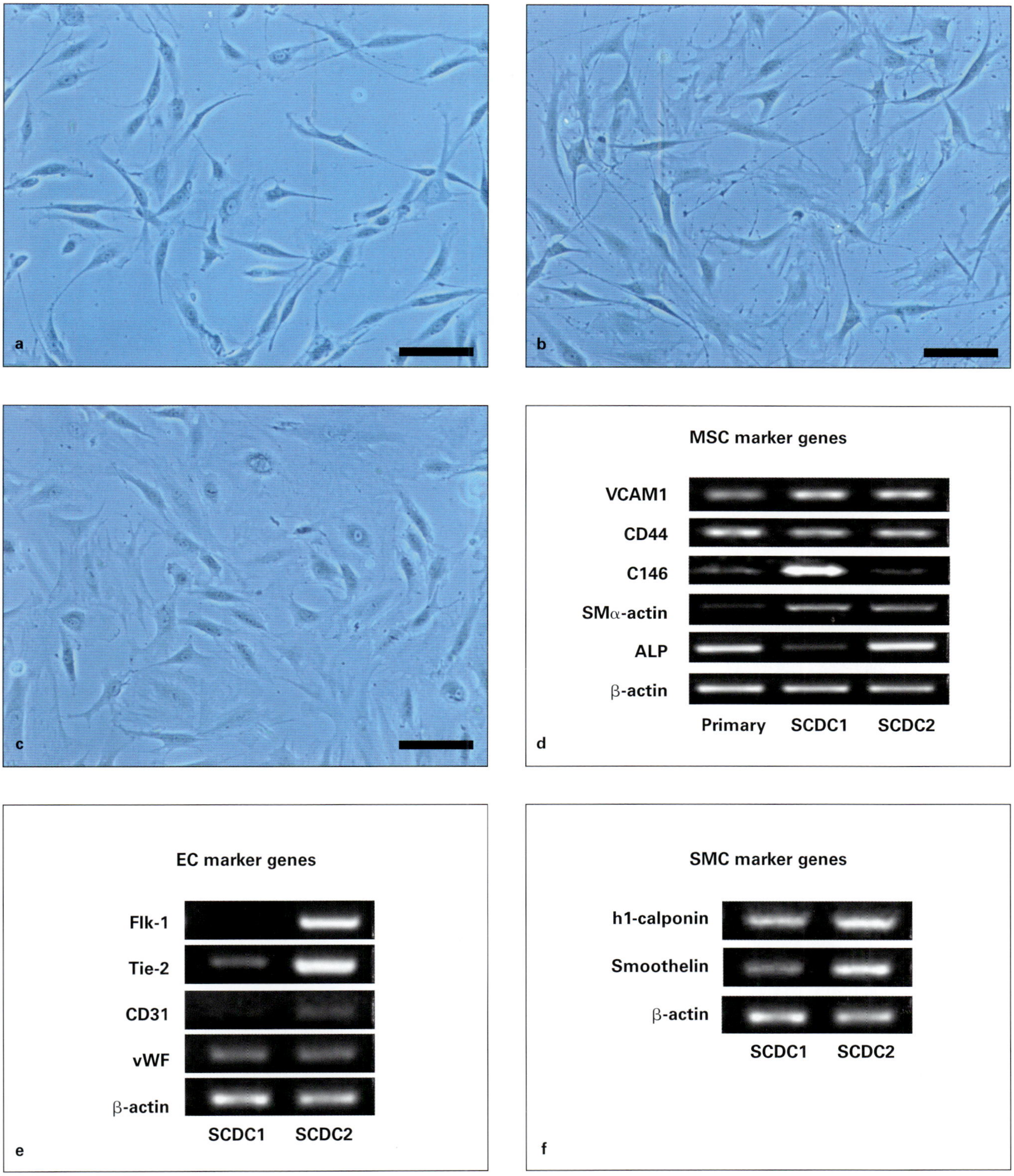

Fig 2-2 Morphologic characterization of rat PDL fibroblasts. *(a to c)* First, rat PDL fibroblasts were cultured on type I collagen–coated plastic plates and viewed by phase-contrast microscopy. Scale bar = 100 µm. *(a)* Primary culture of rat PDL fibroblasts. SCDCs obtained from cultured primary PDL fibroblasts. *(b)* SCDC1. *(c)* SCDC2. *(d to f)* Expression of MSC, EC, and SMC marker genes in rat PDL fibroblasts was determined with reverse-transcriptase polymerase chain reaction using specific primers for genes expressed in MSCs *(d)*, ECs *(e)*, or SMCs *(f)*. Cells obtained from cultured primary rat PDL (primary), SCDC1, and SCDC2 were plated in type I collagen–coated culture dishes. Total cellular RNA was extracted, and the levels of mRNA expression were examined. Equal loading of cDNA samples was confirmed by amplification of β-actin cDNA. VCAM1 = vascular cell adhesion molecule-1; SMα-actin = smooth muscle alpha-actin; ALP = alkaline phosphatase; vWF = von Willebrand factor.

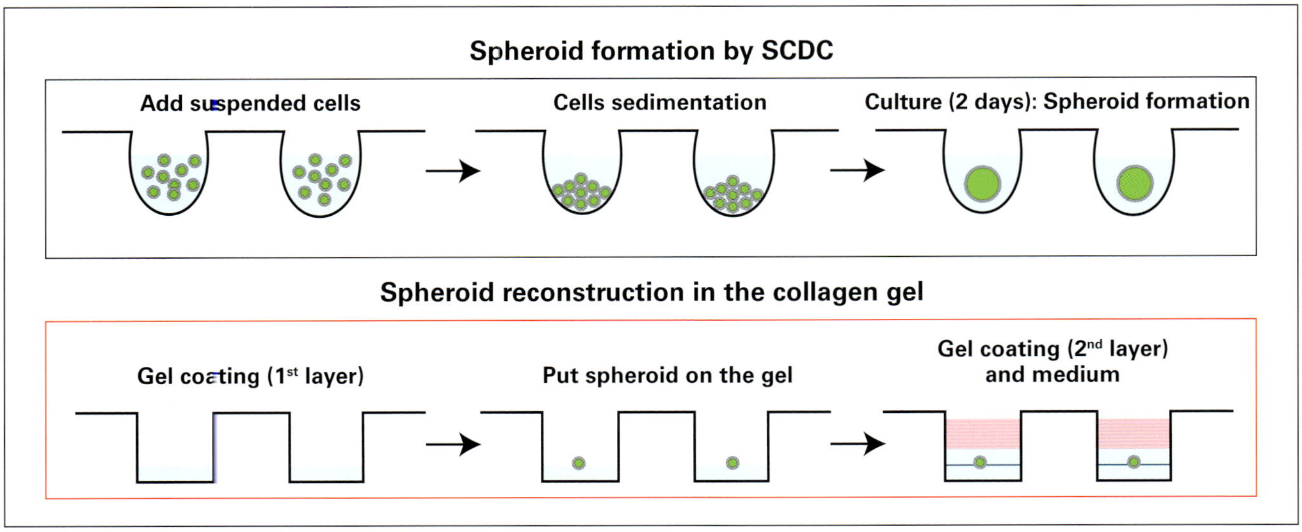

Fig 2-3 Schematic of the three-dimensional culture system.

Reverse-transcriptase polymerase chain reaction (RT-PCR) analysis revealed that the cultured primary PDL fibroblasts and the two types of SCDCs consistently expressed mRNA for MSC markers, ie, CD44, CD146, vascular cell adhesion molecule-1, smooth muscle α-actin, and alkaline phosphatase[19–23] (Fig 2-2d). As shown in Fig 2-2e, mRNA for the EC markers Tie-2, Flk-1, von Willebrand factor, and CD31 was expressed by both SCDCs, although considerable differences were seen in the expression levels of Flk-1, Tie-2, and CD31. In addition, as shown in Fig 2-2f, mRNAs for the SMC markers h1-calponin and smoothelin were consistently expressed in both SCDCs. Thus, SCDCs simultaneously expressed both EC and SMC markers.

Construction of Mature Vessel-like Structures with a Lumen in the Type I Collagen Scaffold by Fibroblasts Derived from PDL

The relationship between the ability of the cells to construct blood vessel structures and the expression of EC markers in PDL fibroblasts was evaluated by comparing SCDC2 with SCDC1. Therefore, the authors evaluated the ability to construct a capillary tubelike structure resembling microvasculature and examined the angiogenic activity of SCDC1 and SCDC2 cells by culturing in a three-dimensional type I collagen scaffold (Fig 2-3).

First, cells were suspended in the culture medium and seeded into a round, nonadhesive plastic plate. The cells were then incubated for 24 hours. During the incubation, the cells migrated toward one another and formed a cluster, resembling a spheroidal aggregation of cells.

This cell cluster was transferred into the type I collagen gel scaffold. Then half of the volume of the gel mixture was pipetted onto the bottom of a well in a 96-well tissue culture plate and incubated to solidify the mixture. After solidification, the spheroidal aggregate of cells constructed was placed onto the center of the solidified gel, and an additional half volume of the type I collagen gel mixture was then placed over the cells and allowed to solidify. Finally, culture medium was added, and the culture was incubated.

As shown in Figs 2-4a and 2-4b, SCDC2 cells constructed many microvasculaturelike structures originating from the entire surface of the spheroidal body. In contrast, SCDC1 cells constructed only a few thin, tubelike structures originating from the loose cell clusters.

Next, expression of a definitive EC marker, Tie-2, was evaluated. The vessel-like structures, composed of SCDC1 and SCDC2 in paraffin-embedded sections, were labeled with anti–Tie-2 polyclonal antibody and phalloidin, which binds cytoskeletal F-actin. No Tie-2 expression was detected in the capillarylike structure in SCDC1 (Fig 2-4c). On the other hand, Tie-2 expression was clearly detected in the vessel-like structure itself or around the edge of the SCDC2 spheroid (Fig 2-4d).

In addition, to investigate the morphologic details of the capillary tubelike structure of SCDC2, celloidin sections (50 µm thick) of SCDC2 in a type I collagen scaffold were obtained and labelled fluorescently using PKH67 Green Fluo-

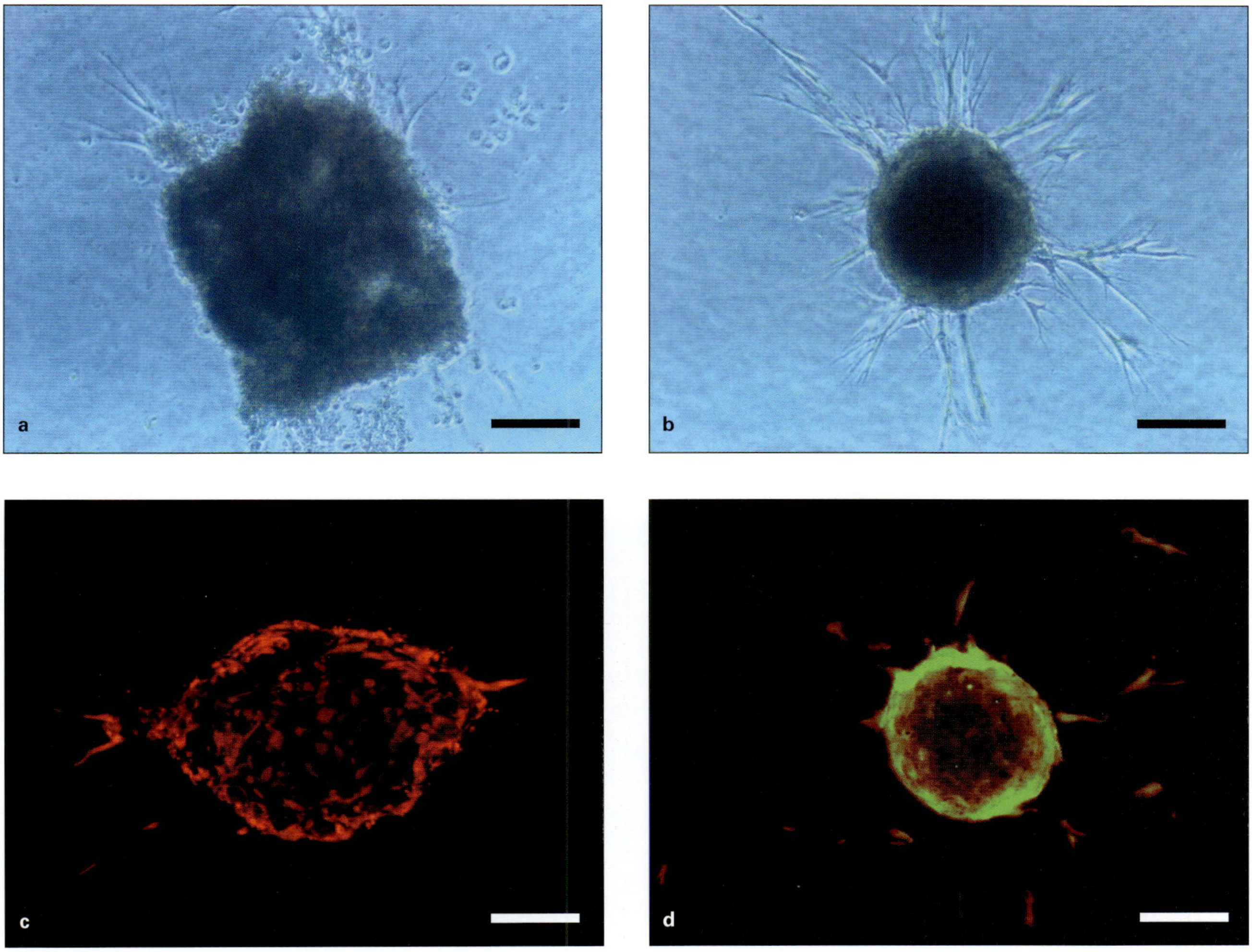

Fig 2-4 Determination of angiogenic activities by culturing SCDCs in a type I collagen scaffold from PDL fibroblasts. Expression in SCDC1 cells *(a)* and SCDC2 cells *(b)*. The SCDC2 cells constructed many microvasculaturelike structures originating from the entire surface of the spheroidal body; in contrast, SCDC1 cells constructed only a few thin, tubelike structures originating from the loose cell clusters. Tie-2 expression is shown for SCDC1 cells *(c)* and SCDC2 cells *(d)*, which were labeled with anti–Tie-2 polydonal antibody *(green)* and phalloidin *(red)*. No Tie-2 expression was seen for SCDC1, but it was clearly detected for SCDC2. Scale bars = 50 µm.

rescent Cell Linker Kit (Sigma-Aldrich). Three-dimensional images of vessel-like structures in celloidin sections were constructed under a fluorescence microscope. Vessel-like structures sprouted from the surface of the spheroidal aggregates (Fig 2-5). Ringlike structures constructed by SCDC2 cells were observed in serial cross sections throughout the vessel-like structure.

Conclusion

Blood vessels are composed of two cell types. ECs line the interior of the vessels, forming channels that allow blood flow, while SMCs cover the outside of vessels, protecting the fragile channels from rupture and controlling blood flow. In this study, SCDC2 cells, which simultaneously express EC and SMC markers (see Figs 2-2e and 2-2f), were shown to have the ability to construct blood vessel-like structures with a mature lumen in a type I collagen gel scaffold.

A sufficient blood supply is indispensable for the regeneration of damaged or lost PDL tissue. An understanding of how PDL tissue recruits precursors of vascular cells and how the precursors differentiate into vascular cells is necessary to establish a practical means of regenerating damaged or lost PDL.

This report has shown that PDL fibroblasts have the potential to show a vascular cell–like ability to construct blood vessel–like structures with a lumen. The authors propose that the fibroblastic lineage in the PDL tissue could be a candidate precursor for construction of a vascular system around damaged PDL tissue to facilitate its regeneration.

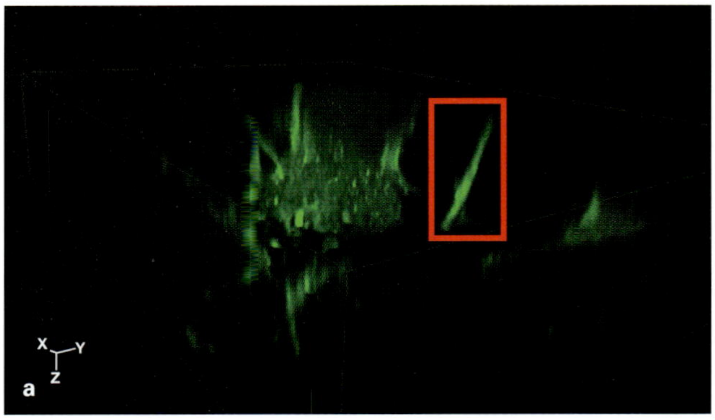

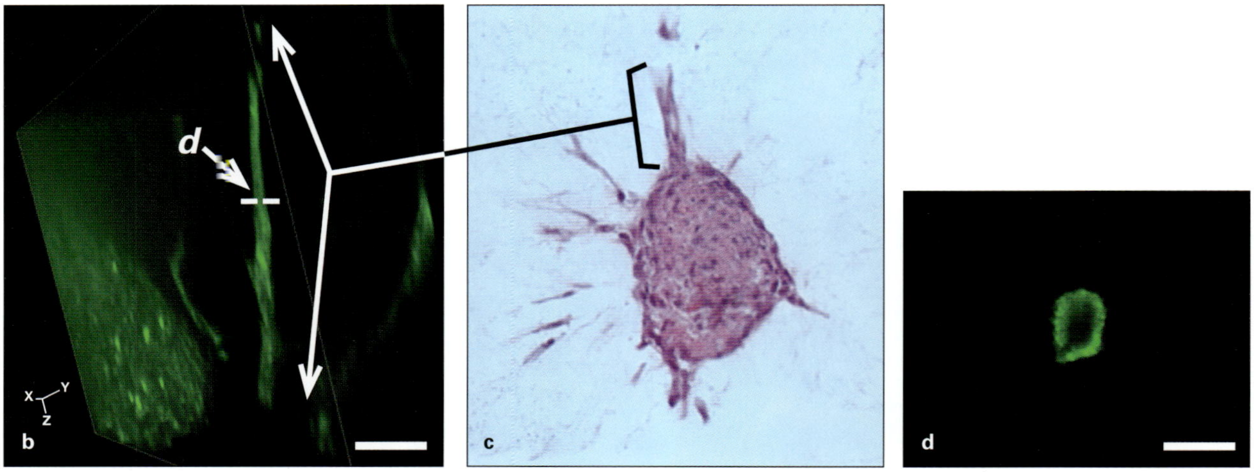

Fig 2-5 Three-dimensional images of the vessel-like structures constructed by SCDC2 cells. *(a)* Vessel-like structures protrude from the surface of the cell cluster. *(b)* Detail of the area enclosed within the *red rectangle* in (a). (Scale bar = 10 μm.) *(c)* Supplementary image corresponding to the vessel-like structures of (b).(Hematoxylin-eosin [HE] staining of paraffin section). *(d)* Ring-like structures constructed by SCDC2 cells observed in a horizontal section indicated by *white arrow* in (b). (Scale bar = 5 μm.)

References

1. Miletich I, Sharpe PT. Neural crest contribution to mammalian tooth formation. Birth Defects Res C Embryo Today 2004;72:200–212.
2. Le Douarin NM, Kalcheim C. The Neural Crest. Cambridge: Cambridge University, 1999.
3. Lekic P, Rojas J, Birek C, Tenenbaum H, McCulloch CA. Phenotypic comparison of periodontal ligament cells in vivo and in vitro. J Periodontal Res 2001;36:71–79.
4. Hammarström L, Heijl L, Gestrelius S. Periodontal regeneration in a buccal dehiscence model in monkeys after application of enamel matrix proteins. J Clin Periodontol 1997;24:669–677.
5. Heijl L, Heden G, Svärdström G, Ostgren A. Enamel matrix derivative (EMDOGAIN) in the treatment of intrabony periodontal defects. J Clin Periodontol 1997;24:705–714.
6. Hammarström L. Enamel matrix, cementum development and regeneration. J Clin Periodontol 1997;24:658–668.
7. Gestrelius S, Andersson C, Lidström D, Hammarström L, Somerman M. In vitro studies on periodontal ligament cells and enamel matrix derivative. J Clin Periodontol 1997;24:685–692.
8. McCulloch CA. Progenitor cell populations in the periodontal ligament of mice. Anat Rec 1985;211:258–262.
9. Pitaru S, Pritzki A, Bar-Kana I, Grosskopf A, Savion N, Narayanan AS. Bone morphogenetic protein 2 induces the expression of cementum attachment protein in human periodontal ligament clones. Connect Tissue Res 2002;43:257–264.
10. Nakamura T, Yamamoto M, Tamura M, Izumi Y. Effects of growth/differentiation factor-5 on human periodontal ligament cells. J Periodontal Res 2003;38:597–605.
11. Trubiani O, Isgro A, Zini N, et al. Functional interleukin-7/interleukin-7Rα, and SDF-1α/CXCR4 are expressed by human periodontal ligament derived mesenchymal stem cells. J Cell Physiol 2008;214:706–713.
12. Shi S, Bartold PM, Miura M, Seo BM, Robey PG, Gronthos S. The efficacy of mesenchymal stem cells to regenerate and repair dental structures. Orthod Craniofac Res 2005;8:191–199.
13. Seo BM, Miura M, Gronthos S, et al. Investigation of multipotent postnatal stem cells from human periodontal ligament. Lancet 2004;364:149–155.
14. Zannettino AC, Roubelakis M, Welldon KJ, et al. Novel mesenchymal and haematopoietic cell isoforms of the SHP-2 docking receptor, PZR: Identification, molecular cloning and effects on cell migration. Biochem J 2003;370:537–549.
15. Bartold PM, Shi S, Gronthos S. Stem cells and periodontal regeneration. Periodontol 2000 2006;40:164–172.
16. Sainz J, Al Haj Zen A, Caligiuri G, et al. Isolation of "side population" progenitor cells from healthy arteries of adult mice. Arterioscler Thromb Vasc Biol 2006;26:281–286.
17. Ishisaki A, Tsunobuchi H, Nakajima K, Imamura T. Possible involvement of protein kinase C activation in differentiation of human umbilical vein endothelium-derived cell into smooth muscle-like cell. Biol Cell 2004;96:499–508.
18. Cevallos M, Riha GM, Wang X, et al. Cyclic strain induces expression of specific smooth muscle cell markers in human endothelial cells. Differentiation 2006;74:552–561.
19. Giannopoulou C, Cimasoni G. Functional characteristics of gingival and periodontal ligament fibroblasts. J Dent Res 1996;75:895–902.
20. Ivanovski S, Gronthos S, Shi S, Bartold PM. Stem cells in the periodontal ligament. Oral Dis 2006;12:358–363.
21. Gronthos S, Mankani M, Brahim J, Robey PG, Shi S. Postnatal human dental pulp stem cells (DPSCs) in vitro and in vivo. Proc Natl Acad Sci U S A 2000;97:13625–13630.
22. Baksh D, Yao R, Tuan RS. Comparison of proliferative and multilineage differentiation potential of human mesenchymal stem cells derived from umbilical cord and bone marrow. Stem Cells 2007;25;1384–1392.
23. Sorrentino A, Ferracin M, Castelli G, et al. Isolation and characterization of CD146+ multipotent mesenchymal stromal cells. Exp Hematol 2008;36:1035–1046.

3

Gene Expression of BMP Receptor and Osteopontin in In Vitro–Induced Odontoblast-like Cells

Masaru Murata, Youssef Haikel, Hervé Lesot, Jean Victor Ruch, Hidetsugu Tsujigiwa, Makato Arisue, Noriyuki Nagai

The developing tooth is an interesting model in which to study the molecular mechanisms involved in the epithelial-mesenchymal interactions controlling histomorphogenesis and cytodifferentiation.[1–3] In the mandibular first molar in the mouse, a terminal differentiation of odontoblasts occurs at the late bell stage (embryonic days 18 to 20). Terminal differentiation is characterized by action of the preodontoblasts: They withdraw from the cell cycle, polarize, and secrete predentin-dentin components, including collagen, phosphophoryn, dentin matrix protein-1, and dentin sialoprotein.[4] When dental papillae are isolated by treatment with proteolytic enzymes and either cultured in vitro or grafted in vivo, preodontoblasts never differentiate.[5,6] Specific epigenetic signals trigger odontoblast terminal differentiation. Previous studies have shown that bone morphogenetic protein 2 (BMP-2), BMP-4, osteonectin, and bone sialoprotein transcripts were detected in odontoblasts during tooth development[7,8] and, in vitro, in induced odontoblast-like cells.[2,9] To better understand the roles of BMPs and osteopontin (OPN), the authors investigated the mRNA expression of both BMP receptors and OPN in a dental papillae culture model.

Materials and Methods

Removal of tooth germ and isolation of dental papillae

Swiss mice in day 17 of pregnancy (vaginal plug day = day 0) were sacrificed by cervical dislocation. The embryos were removed, and the mandibular first molars were isolated. The day-17 tooth germs were incubated for 45 minutes at 4°C in 1% trypsin in Hank's solution, and enamel organs and dental papillae were enzymatically dissociated with the trypsin solution.[9] Isolated dental papillae were immersed twice in fetal calf serum/Hank's solution (1:1 ratio by volume) to inhibit the activity of the enzyme.

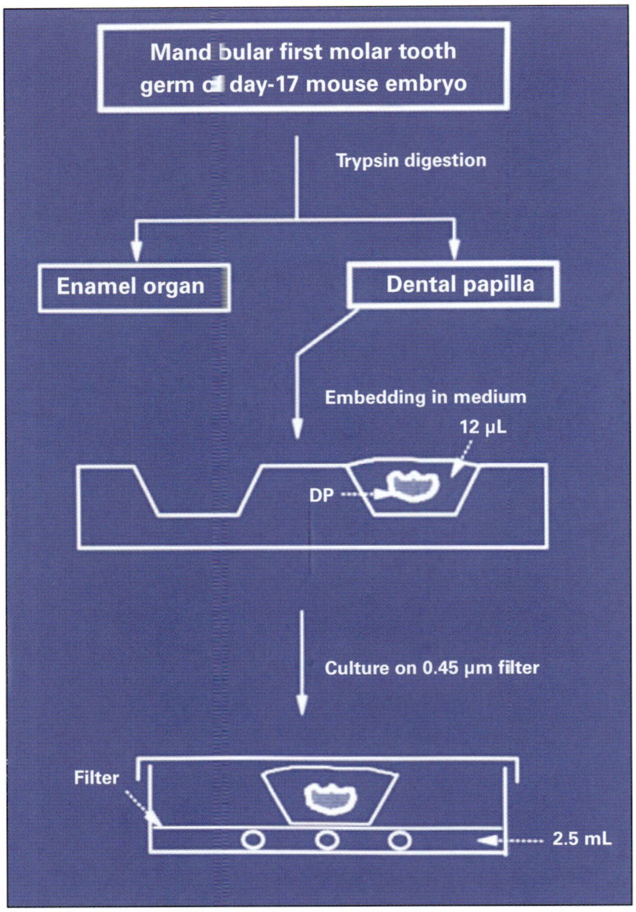

Fig 3-1 Protocol for dental papilla (DP) culture. The DP was mechanically separated from the enamel organ after trypsin dissociation of tooth germs and embedded in 12 µL of semisolid medium. The dental papilla embedded in the semisolid medium was deposited on Millipore filters and cultured for 6 days in Trowell-type culture in the presence of 2.5 mL of liquid medium at 37°C in 95% air and 5% carbon dioxide. The liquid medium was changed every 2 days.

Preparation of BMP solution

BMPs were partially purified from bovine cortical bone and characterized biochemically. The BMP fraction contained BMP-2 and contaminants such as histones H3 and H2B and was free of basic fibroblast growth factor and transforming growth factor-ß1 and -ß2. The BMP fraction was dissolved in 4 mmol/L hydrochloric acid, and the BMP solutions were prepared at determined concentrations as follows: BMPs alone (0.5, 1.0, 2.0, 4.0 µg/µL) and BMPs mixed with heparin (0.5, 1.0, or 2.0 µg/µL) containing 1.2 µg of heparin (Sigma) in 2 µL of solution. For the combination solution, BMP solution and heparin solution were mixed and incubated for 1 hour at 4°C before use.

Tissue culture

The dental papillae were embedded individually in 10 µL of culture medium composed of BGJ-b medium, ascorbic acid (0.18 mg/mL), L-glutamine (2 mmol/L), kanamycin (0.1 mg/mL), fetal calf serum (20%), and agar (0.5%). Then 2 µL of each BMP solution were added to the medium before gelling. The dental papillae embedded in the semisolid medium were deposited on Millipore filters and cultured for 6 days in Trowell-type culture in the presence of 2.5 mL of liquid control medium at 37°C in 95% air and 5% carbon dioxide. The liquid medium was changed every 2 days (Fig 3-1). The dose response and the time course for 6- and 10-day studies of odontoblast-like cell differentiation by BMPs were investigated in this culture model.

Histologic observations

Tissues were fixed in Bouin's solution and stained with Mallory's Alun hematoxylin or in 4% paraformaldehyde for in situ hybridization. The fixed tissues were embedded in paraffin and cut serially. Sections 5 µm in thickness were stained with Mallory's Alun hematoxylin. In addition, digoxigenin-labeled cRNA probes were prepared from mouse BMP receptor cDNA (the product displays specific binding to BMP-2 and BMP-4 and OPN cDNA using the DIG-RNA Labeling Kit and Dig Nucleic Acid Detection Kit [Boehringer]).

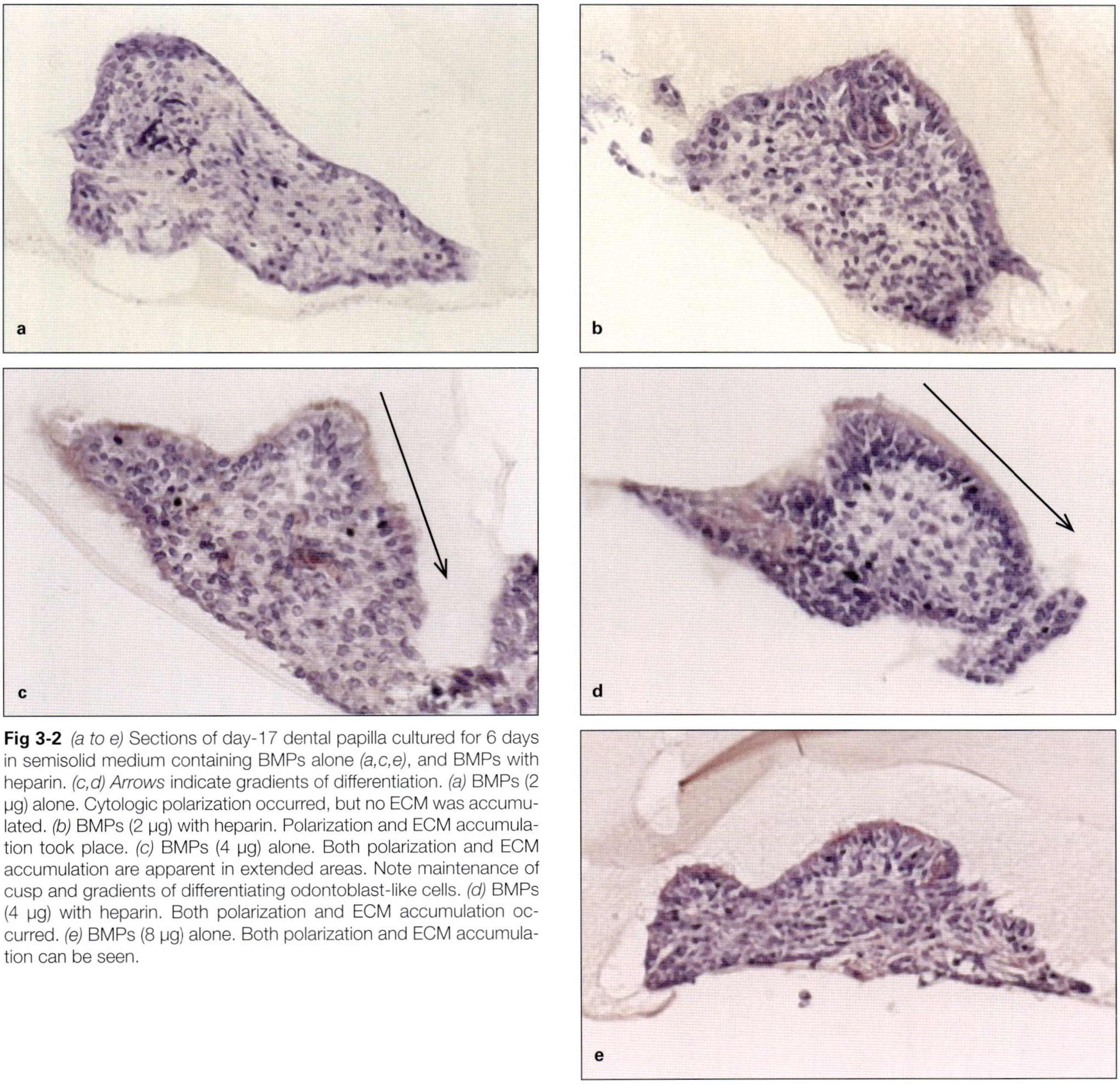

Fig 3-2 *(a to e)* Sections of day-17 dental papilla cultured for 6 days in semisolid medium containing BMPs alone *(a,c,e)*, and BMPs with heparin. *(c,d) Arrows* indicate gradients of differentiation. *(a)* BMPs (2 µg) alone. Cytologic polarization occurred, but no ECM was accumulated. *(b)* BMPs (2 µg) with heparin. Polarization and ECM accumulation took place. *(c)* BMPs (4 µg) alone. Both polarization and ECM accumulation are apparent in extended areas. Note maintenance of cusp and gradients of differentiating odontoblast-like cells. *(d)* BMPs (4 µg) with heparin. Both polarization and ECM accumulation occurred. *(e)* BMPs (8 µg) alone. Both polarization and ECM accumulation can be seen.

Results and Discussion

The induction of cytologic polarization and apical extracellular matrix (ECM) accumulation were dependent on the dose (0, 1, 2, 4, 8 µg) of exogenous BMPs in papillae cultured in vitro for 6 days (Figs 3-2a to 3-2e). (Note the negative control in Fig 3-2f.) In situ hybridization indicated that BMP receptor mRNA was distributed in odontoblast-like/preodontoblast-like cells (Fig 3-2g) and OPN mRNA was uniquely detected in odontoblast-like cells (Fig 3-2h). BMP receptor and OPN mRNA were codistributed in odontoblast-like cells. Integration of these data with previous works suggests that endogenous BMP-2 and BMP-4 produced by odontoblasts should act as an autocrine/paracrine mediator in tooth development. Moreover, OPN should be one of the marker proteins for odontoblast terminal differentiation.

These results demonstrate that, in the presence of BMP-2 and other components, even without heparin, the initiation of odontoblast differentiation with maintenance of physiologic gradients can be obtained, despite the absence of an inner dental epithelium and a competent basement membrane. The present observations indicate that BMP-2 stimulated the cytologic and functional differentiation of preodontoblasts and also that other components (except for heparin) might play important roles as substrates and/or synergistic cofactors of BMP-2.

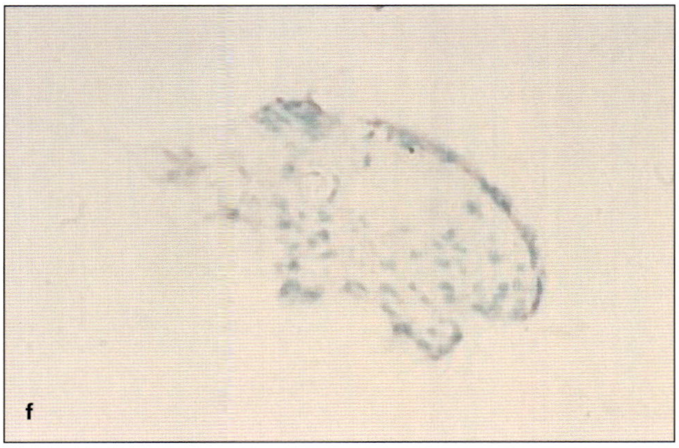

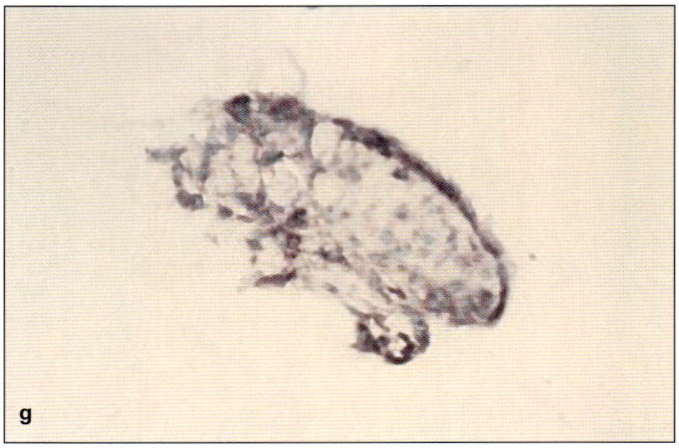

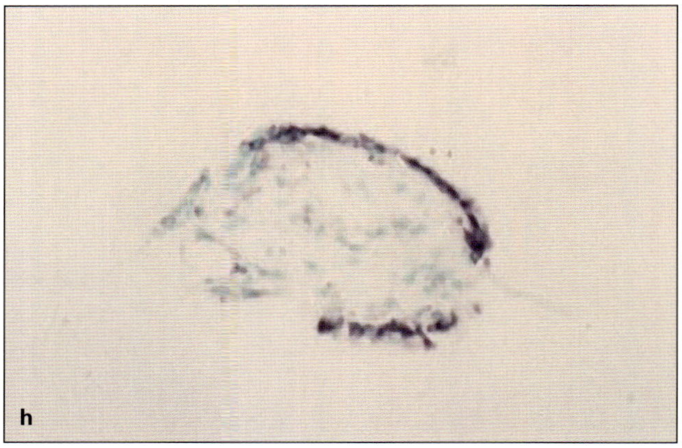

Fig 3-2 *(cont) (f to h)* Gene expression of BMP receptor and OPN in day-17 dental papilla cultured for 6 days in semisolid medium containing 2 µg of BMPs with heparin. *(f)* Negative control with neither BMPs nor herparin. *(g)* BMP receptor mRNA distributed in odontoblast-like/preodontoblast-like cells. *(h)* OPN mRNA was uniquely detected in odontoblast-like cells at the periphery of the papillae. Note the codistribution of both BMP receptor and OPN mRNA in odontoblast-like cells.

References

1. Ruch JV. Tooth crown morphogenesis and cytodifferentiations: Candid questions and critical comments. Connect Tissue Res 1995;31:1–8.
2. Ruch JV, Lesot H, Begue-Kirn C. Odontoblast differentiation. Int J Dev Biol 1995;39:51–68.
3. Thesleff I, Vaahtokari A, Partanen AM. Regulation of organogenesis. Common molecular mechanisms regulating the development of teeth and other organs. Int J Dev Biol 1995;39:35–50.
4. Butler TK, Ritchie H. The nature and functional significance of dentin extracellular matrix proteins. Int J Dev Biol 1995;39:169–179.
5. Osman M, Ruch JV. Behavior of odontoblasts and basal lamina of trypsin or EDTA-isolated mouse dental papillae in short-term culture. J Dent Res 1981;60:1015–1027.
6. Ruch JV. Odontoblast differentiation and the formation of the odontoblast layer. J Dent Res 1985;64:480–488.
7. Vainio S, Karavanova I, Jowett A, Thesleff I. Identification of BMP-4 as a signal mediating secondary induction between epithelial and mesenchymal tissues during early tooth development. Cell 1993;75:45–58.
8. Heikinheimo K. Stage-specific expression of decapentaplegic-Vg-related genes 2, 4, and 6 (bone morphogenetic proteins 2, 4, and 6) during human tooth morphogenesis. J Dent Res 1994;73:590–595.
9. Bègue-Kirn C, Smith AJ, Loriot M, Kupferle C, Ruch JV, Lesot H. Comparative analysis of TGFβs, BMPs, IGF1, msxs, fibronectin, osteonectin and bone sialoprotein gene expression during normal and in vitro-induced odontoblast differentiation. Int J Dev Biol 1994;38:405–420.

4

Dentin Conditioning with BMP for Reconstruction of Periodontal Attachment

Hirofumi Miyaji, Masamitsu Kawanami

Periodontitis refers to inflammation of the supporting structures of the teeth and is associated with loss of periodontal tissues, eg, periodontal membrane, cementum, and alveolar bone. Most cases of periodontitis involve microbial infections and result in deep periodontal pockets. Therefore, the objectives of periodontal therapy are to remove the pathogenic bacteria and contaminated cementum from the pocket and to regenerate the periodontal attachment to the root dentin surface. However, it is difficult to achieve these objectives because regeneration of the attachment is prevented by the rapid downgrowth of the junctional epithelium along the root surface and formation of gingival connective tissue, which has few osteogenic cells, during the early stages of healing.

Dentin consists of approximately 75% inorganic material, 20% organic material, and 5% other constituents. It has a unique structure, with numerous dentinal tubules extending across its entire width. Agents used for dentin demineralization remove the surface smear layer, open the dentinal tubules, and expose the organic elements, such as collagen matrix, thus increasing its total surface area (Fig 4-1). The extracellular matrix is an attractive target for locally applied therapeutic agents. It has been suggested that demineralized dentin provides a suitable surface for the retention of bioactive substances, such as growth factors and local drug delivery agents, in regenerative therapy.

Various growth factors have been used in periodontal tissue engineering. Bone morphogenetic proteins (BMPs) are known to promote the mineralization of nonosteogenic cells and formation of bone.[1,2] Since BMPs have the ability to bind to the collagen matrix, demineralized dentin might serve as a suitable carrier of BMPs. It was reported that dentin treated with both ethylenediaminetetraacetic acid (EDTA) and BMP stimulated the osteogenic activity of periodontal ligament (PDL) cells attached to dentin.[3] Therefore, root dentin conditioning with BMPs may promote the formation of cementumlike tissue on the dentin, resulting in early establishment of a stable attachment between the root dentin and gingival connective tissue during initial periodontal wound healing.

This chapter describes two experiments conducted in animal models to evaluate surface treatment with BMPs. The purpose of these investigations was to determine the effect of dentin conditioning with BMPs on periodontal wound healing and periodontal reattachment.

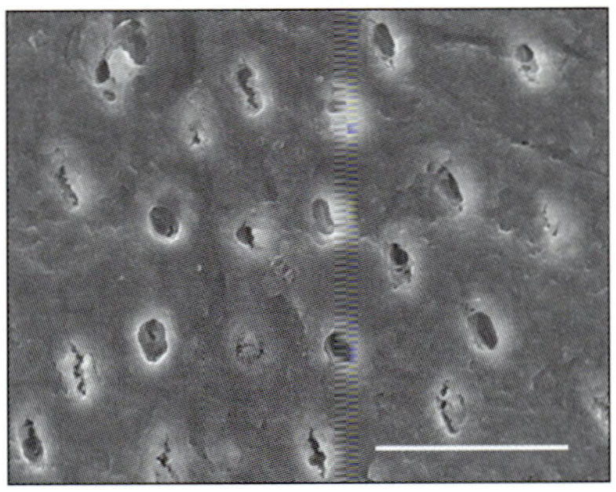

Fig 4-1 Scanning electron microscopic image of a demineralized dentin surface. The cross sections of dentinal tubules have been exposed by treatment with ethylenediaminetetraacetic acid. Intertubular dentin matrix can be seen on the denuded dentin surface. Scale bar = 10 µm.

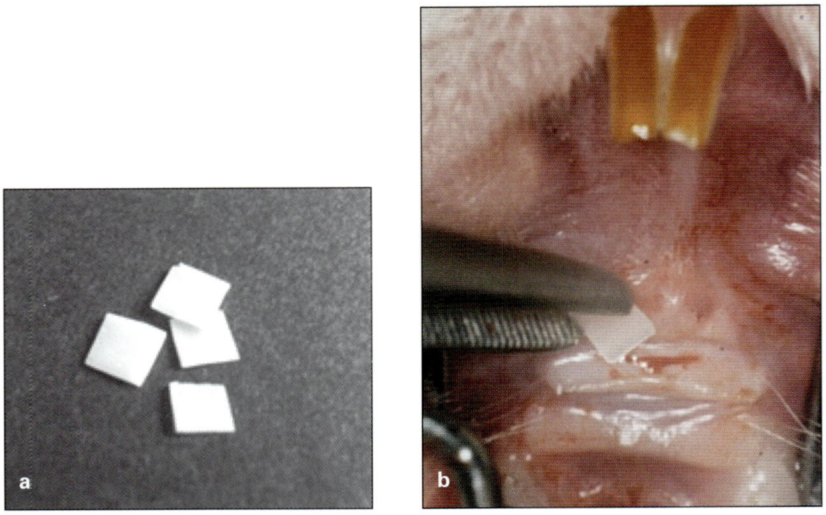

Fig 4-2 *(a)* Dentin blocks prepared from rat root dentin. *(b)* The block, treated with BMP, was implanted in rat palatal connective tissue.

Dentin Conditioning with BMPs for the Reconstruction of Cementum in Rats

Dentin blocks treated with different doses of BMPs were prepared, and these were implanted in rat palatal connective tissue.[4,5] This model examined the dose-related tissue responses of BMPs on the dentin surface.

Materials and methods

Flat dentin blocks were prepared from rat root dentin and treated for 3 minutes with EDTA (Fig 4-2a). These blocks were then immersed in recombinant human BMP-2 solution (0.1 or 0.4 mg/mL, Astellas Pharmaceutical) for 10 minutes. As a control, dentin blocks were treated with phosphate-buffered saline alone.

Wistar rats (10 weeks old) were used in this experiment. With the animals under general and local anesthesia, the BMP-conditioned dentin blocks were implanted into the connective tissue of the masticatory mucosa of the hard palate (Fig 4-2b).

Specimens were prepared 2 and 8 weeks after surgery. Serial paraffin sections were prepared and stained with hematoxylin-eosin (HE) and tartrate-resistant acid phosphatase (TRAP). Osteocalcin immunolocalization was also performed.

Results

In the control blocks, no attachment with formation of cementum or PDL was observed on the dentin surfaces at any experimental stage.

In contrast, in test specimens, deposits of cementumlike tissue were demonstrated on dentin (Figs 4-3a and 4-3b). The cementumlike tissue layer was thin, with irregular areas of thickness, and included cementocytelike cells, which were attached to the connective tissue. However, there were no insertions of collagen fibers such as Sharpey's fibers, and no PDL-like structures had formed. Dentin resorption was also clearly observed. New cementumlike tissue had randomly formed on parts of the nonresorbed and resorbed dentin surfaces. Osteocalcin was noted around the cementoblast cells, lining the surface of the cementumlike tissue (Fig 4-3c).

In specimens immersed in high doses of BMPs, obvious dentin resorption by osteoclastic cells was frequently observed on the dentin surface (Fig 4-3d). New cementumlike tissue had formed poorly on the dentin. Resorbed areas showed some resorption lacunae associated with TRAP-positive cells (Figs 4-3e and 4-3f).

Discussion

It has been reported that BMPs stimulate bone formation in the body. However, interestingly, cementumlike tissue was also formed on the dentin in the present study, suggesting that mineralized tissue formation on the dentin surface was

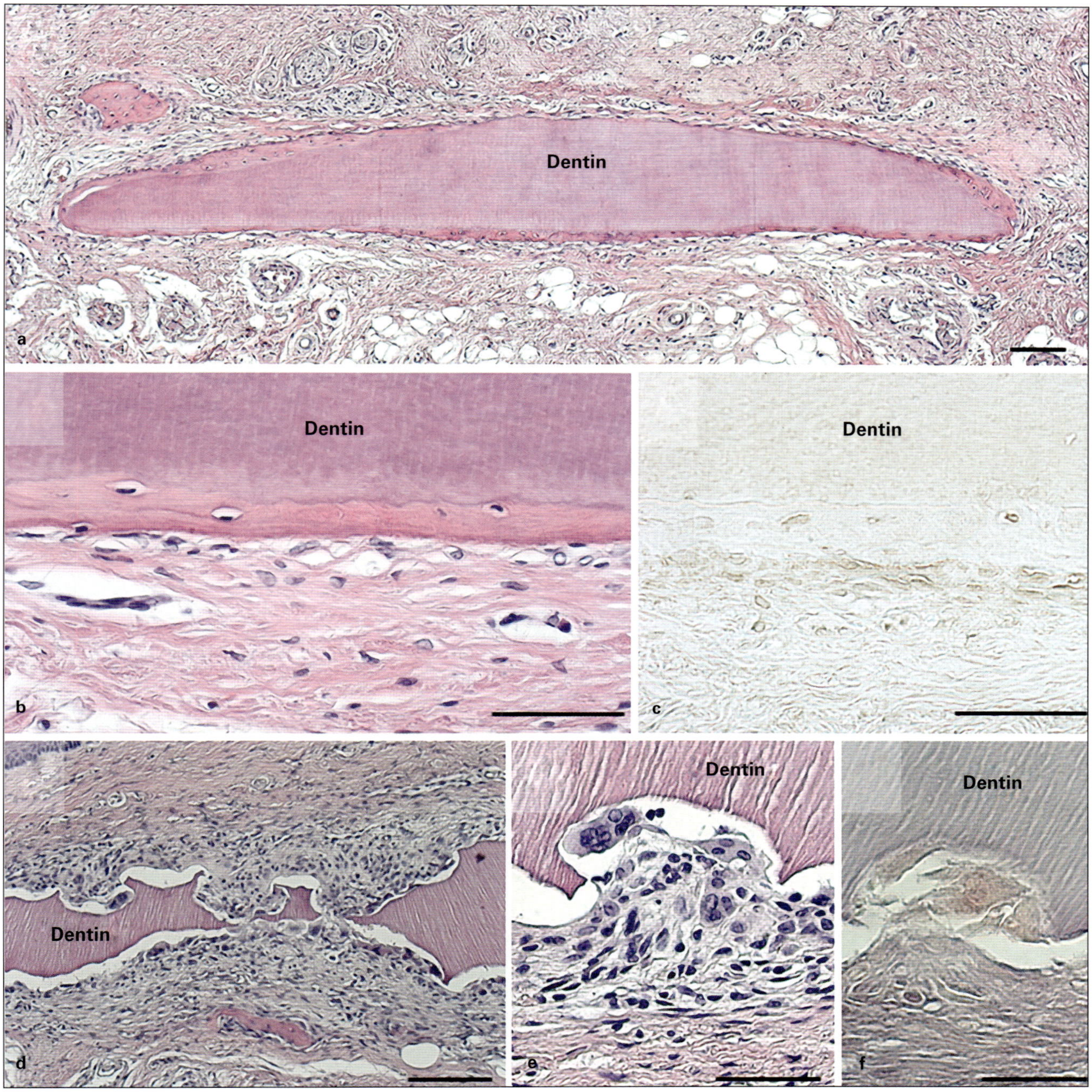

Fig 4-3 Light micrographs demonstrating implanted dentin blocks after 8 weeks of treatment (HE *[a to e]*, TRAP *[f]*; scale bars = 100 µm *(a,d)* and 50 µm *(b,c,e,f)*. *(a)* Dentin block treated with BMP at 0.1 µg/µL. New cementumlike tissue had formed on the dentin surface. *(b)* The cementumlike tissue layer was thin and included cementocytelike cells. *(c)* Osteocalcin was noted around the cementoblastic cells, lining the surface of the newly formed cementumlike tissue. *(d)* Dentin block treated with BMP at 0.4 µg/µL. BMP loading at a high dose facilitated dentin resorption. *(e,f)* Resorption lacunae were associated with giant cells, which were TRAP positive.

strongly associated with extracellular matrix of dentin and/or dentin surface morphology. Dentin may play a key role in cementogenesis following BMP surface treatment. On the other hand, cementumlike tissue formed on resorbed and/or nonresorbed dentin surfaces after treatment with BMP. From this evidence, the authors speculate that two different biologic mechanisms are involved in BMP conditioning leading to cementumlike tissue formation: *(1)* BMPs directly regulate osteoblastic differentiation of undifferentiated mesenchymal cells in connective tissue, and *(2)* osteoclastic cell–based remodeling associated with BMP application augments reparative cementum deposition. In periodontal wound healing, a remodeling process with osteoclastic resorption and deposition of repair cementum is generally seen on the root surface, leading to regeneration of the periodontal attachment.

Table 4-1 **Histomorphometric findings at 2 and 8 weeks after surgery**

	Control		0.1 µg/µL BMP		0.4 µg/µL BMP	
	2 wk	8 wk	2 wk	8 wk	2 wk	8 wk
Cementumlike tissue (%)	0.0 ± 0.0	0.0 ± 0.0	3.5 ± 4.7*	41.8 ± 18.3*	6.7± 8.9*	16.2 ± 20.3*†
Resorbed dentin area (%)	1.1 ± 1.9	1.1 ± 1.7	2.0 ± 1.8*	4.9 ± 3.7*	5.0 ± 2.8*†	14.4 ± 9.0*†

Means ± standard deviations shown; n = 8 per group. Cementumlike tissue is the percentage of the length of the newly formed cementumlike tissue to the length of the total dentin block surface. Resorbed dentin is the percentage of the resorbed dentin area to the total dentin block area. Differences among groups were analyzed using the modified Mann-Whitney *U* test. $P < .05$ was considered statistically significant.
*Statistically significant difference compared with control group. †Statistically significant difference compared with 0.1 µg/µL BMP application group.

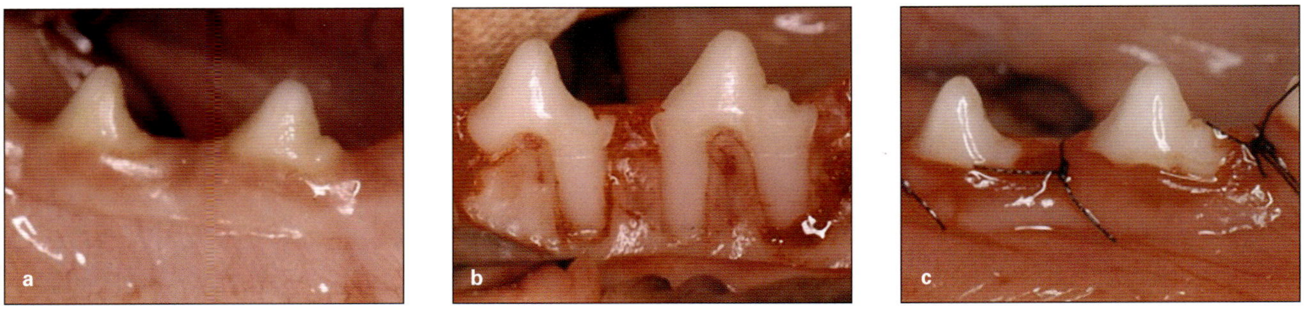

Fig 4-4 *(a)* Preoperative view of the experimental area. *(b)* Dehiscence-type periodontal defects were created. *(c)* After BMPs were applied to the root dentin surface, the flaps were repositioned and sutured.

Application of BMPs caused a dose-related increase in dentin resorption; however, the osteogenic effect of BMPs was inversely dose-dependent (Table 4-1). Recent studies using dentin pit resorption assay have demonstrated that BMP-2 significantly stimulated osteoclast differentiation and osteoclast resorption activity.[6,7] Therefore, dentin resorption is conceivably modulated by variations in the dosage of BMP. Some investigators reported that in vitro bioactivities of cells were accelerated by optimal concentration of growth factors but inhibited by higher concentrations.[8] Thus, application of a BMP overdose (0.4 mg/mL) in rats may inhibit cementumlike tissue formation. Dentin surface conditioning with appropriate doses of BMPs may enhance the predictable formation of new periodontal attachment to dentin.

Influence of Root Dentin Modification with BMPs on Periodontal Wound Healing in Dogs

The purpose of this study was to examine whether root dentin modification with BMPs would induce cementumlike tissue deposition in experimental periodontal defects in beagle dogs.[9,10] This study also investigated the effect of BMP application on periodontal wound healing.

Materials and methods

Beagle dogs, 10 to 12 months old, were used in this experiment. Surgical procedures were performed under general and local anesthesia. After a gingival flap was elevated on the buccal side of the maxillary and mandibular premolars, alveolar bone was removed to a depth of 6 mm with a rotating round bur. The root surface was planed to remove cementum.[11] Subsequently, the denuded dentin was demineralized with EDTA for 3 minutes. Fifteen µL of BMP-2 solution (0.4 and 1.0 mg/mL) was applied to the root dentin by pipette and acrylic resin sponge. As a control, phosphate-buffered saline alone was applied to the dentin. The flap was repositioned and securely sutured (Fig 4-4).

Specimens were collected from the wounds at 16 weeks postsurgery. The tissue blocks were fixed and embedded in paraffin wax. Serial sections were prepared and stained with HE.

Results and discussion

In the control specimens, gingival connective tissue was seen attached to the root dentin in most areas. There was no cementumlike tissue on the dentin surface. Downgrowth of the junctional epithelium was frequently observed in the coronal portion. There was no ankylosis, but mild induction of bone was noted (Fig 4-5a).

In contrast, in the BMP-treated specimens, new cementumlike tissue had been deposited on the dentin (Figs 4-5b

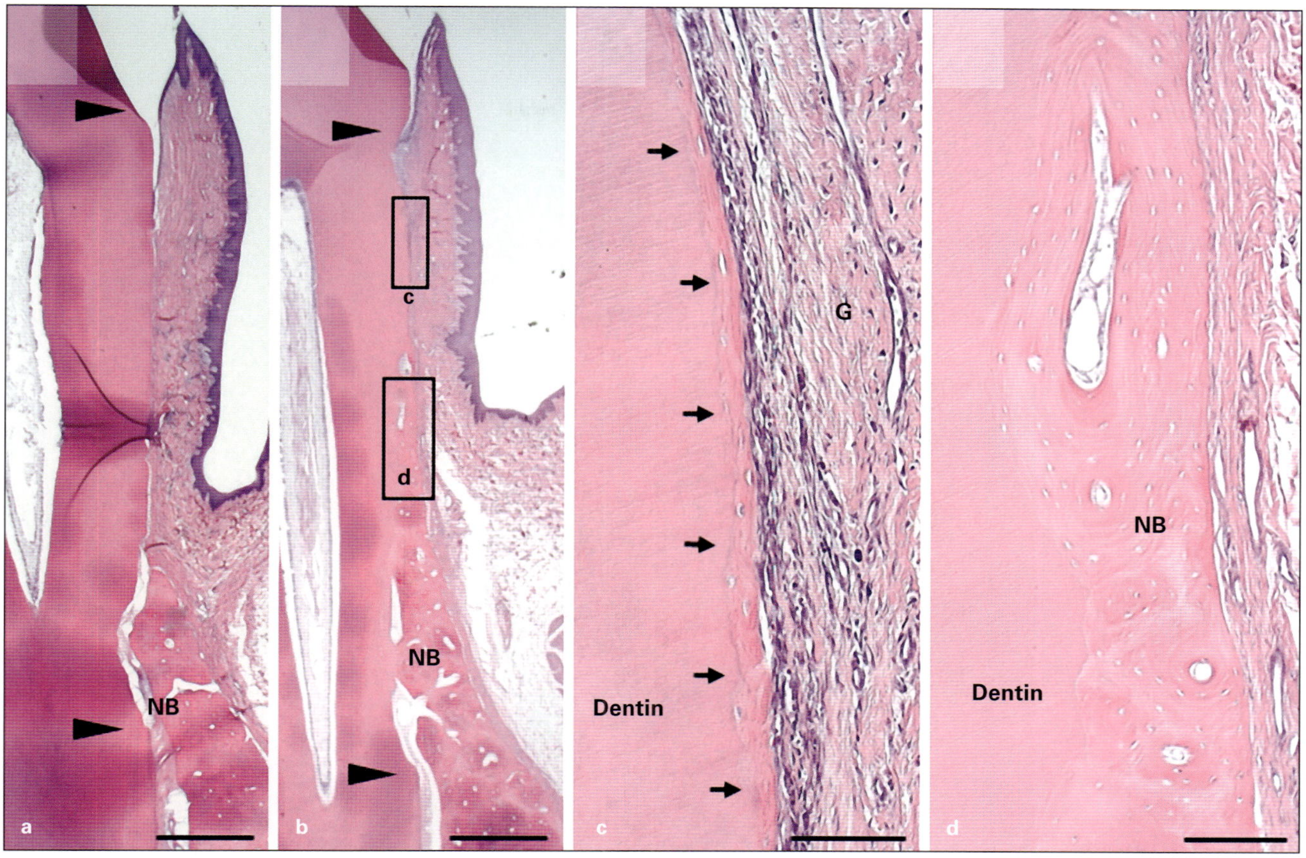

Fig 4-5 Histologic findings in control and BMP-treated specimens in beagle dogs (HE; scale bars = 1 mm *[a,b]*, 100 µm *[c]*, and 200 µm *[d]*). *Arrowheads* indicate coronal and apical notches. *(a)* Histologic findings in control specimen. Gingival connective tissue was attached to the root dentin surface without bone and cementum formation. New bone (NB) was seen only in the apical portion of the defect. *(b)* Histologic findings in the group treated with BMPs at 1.0 µg/µL. Gingival connective tissue is attached to the root surface, and new bone formation has been induced at the apical end of the site. *(c)* Higher-magnification view of the smaller framed area in *(b)*. Cellular cementumlike tissue *(arrows)* was frequently detected on the BMP-conditioned root dentin surface, covered by gingival connective tissue (G). *(d)* Higher-magnification view of the larger outlined area in *(b)*. Ankylosis and root dentin resorption have accelerated in the defect area.

Table 4-2 **Histomorphometric findings at 16 weeks after surgery**

	Control (n = 8)	0.4 µg/µL BMP (n = 6)	1.0 µg/µL BMP (n = 7)
Cementumlike tissue (%)	0.0 ± 0.0	8.1 ± 5.5	39.0 ± 31.9*†
New bone (%)	37.7 ± 12.6	55.1 ± 13.3	65.4 ± 16.6*

Means ± standard deviations shown. Cementumlike tissue volume is the percentage of the length of the newly formed cementumlike tissue to the length of the attached gingival connective tissue. New bone is the percentage of the length of the newly formed alveolar bone to the defect height. Differences among the groups were analyzed using the Scheffé test. $P < .05$ was considered statistically significant.
*Statistically significant difference compared with control group. †Statistically significant difference compared with the 0.4 µg/µL BMP application group.

and 4-5c). Thick cementumlike cellular tissue with a layered appearance, ie, a cement line, resembling cellular intrinsic fiber cementum was frequently seen. Cementumlike deposits were lined by cementoblastlike cells and attached to gingival connective tissue. However, Sharpey's fibers were not detected, as in the aforementioned rat study. Downgrowth of the junctional epithelium was suppressed at the coronal portion of the root. In the apical portion of the BMP application group, new alveolar bone had also formed; however, ankylosis with dentin resorption was also seen (Fig 4-5d). A PDL space between the alveolar bone and root surface was evident; however, the cells and extracellular matrix were poorly distributed at the interface. Osteoclastic cells were predominant in the ankylotic sites.

Histomorphometric measurements were performed for each stained section (Table 4-2). There was a BMP dose–dependent increase in the amount of cementumlike tissue and bone.

Histologic findings revealed that BMP surface treatment of the dentin frequently caused deposition of cementumlike tissue encapsulated within gingival connective tissue. These results support the notion that restoration of a stable periodontal attachment can be guided on the root surface regardless of whether original PDL tissues remain. It seems likely that the only remaining cell source is the gingival connective tissue when the surgical flap is reattached to the instrumented dentin surface in cases of advanced periodontitis.

BMP treatment consistently resulted in alveolar bone induction. It has been suggested that alveolar bone formation was augmented by BMPs released from the dentin in this therapy. However, application of high doses of BMPs induced ankylosis and root resorption. Ankylosis was evident in five of the six defect sites that received BMP at 0.4 mg/mL and at all seven roots treated at a dose of 1.0 mg/mL. The authors believe that the root resorption and ankylosis would be inhibited by regeneration of the PDL in periodontal regenerative therapy. However, the present study also showed that reestablishment of the PDL was poor. BMP-2 has demonstrated low proliferative activity on human PDL cells in vitro.[3] Thus, BMP-2 localized on the dentin surface would suppress the proliferation of PDL cells in early periodontal wound healing. To prevent ankylosis with a BMP conditioning system, additional steps may be necessary to accelerate the biologic activities of PDL cells. Aberrations resulting from BMP use must be verified in the future.

Conclusions

Dentin conditioning with BMPs plays a significant role in promoting cementumlike tissue formation on instrumented dentin. Therefore, dentin biomodification by BMP application may allow reestablishment of periodontal attachment in case of advanced periodontal destruction, regardless of the source of the cells provided to the dentin surface.

References

1. Barr T, McNamara AJ, Sándor GK, Clokie CM, Peel SA. Comparison of the osteoinductivity of bioimplants containing recombinant human bone morphogenetic proteins 2 (Infuse) and 7 (OP-1). Oral Surg Oral Med Oral Pathol Oral Radiol Endod 2010;109:531–540.
2. Inoue K, Miyaji H, Sugaya T, Kawanami M. Ectopic bone induction by BMP-loaded collagen scaffold and bone marrow stromal cell sheet. J Oral Tissue Eng 2010;8:19–29.
3. Zaman KU, Sugaya T, Kato H. Effect of recombinant human platelet-derived growth factor-BB and bone morphogenetic protein-2 application to demineralized dentin on early periodontal ligament cell response. J Periodontal Res 1999;34:244–250.
4. Miyaji H, Sugaya T, Miyamoto T, Kato K, Kato H. Hard tissue formation on dentin surfaces applied with recombinant human bone morphogenetic protein-2 in the connective tissue of the palate. J Periodontal Res 2002;37:204–209.
5. Miyaji H, Sugaya T, Kato K, Kawamura N, Tsuji H, Kawanami M. Dentin resorption and cementum-like tissue formation by bone morphogenetic protein application. J Periodontal Res 2006;41:311–315.
6. Kaneko H, Arakawa T, Mano H, et al. Direct stimulation of osteoclastic bone resorption by bone morphogenetic protein (BMP)-2 and expression of BMP receptors in mature osteoclasts. Bone 2000;27:479–486.
7. Jensen ED, Pham L, Billington CJ Jr, et al. Bone morphogenic protein 2 directly enhances differentiation of murine osteoclast precursors. J Cell Biochem 2010;109:672–682.
8. Nishimura F, Terranova VP. Comparative study of the chemotactic responses of periodontal ligament cells and gingival fibroblasts to polypeptide growth factors. J Dent Res 1996;75:986–992.
9. Miyaji H, Sugaya T, Ibe K, Ishizuka R, Tokunaga K, Kawanami M. Root surface conditioning with bone morphogenetic protein-2 facilitates cementum-like tissue deposition in beagle dogs. J Periodontal Res 2010;45:658–663.
10. Miyaji H, Sugaya T, Ibe K, Ishizuka R, Tokunaga K, Kawanami M. Influence of root surface conditioning with bone morphogenetic protein-2 on periodontal wound healing in beagle dogs. J Oral Tissue Eng 2011;8:173–180.
11. Miyaji H, Sugaya T, Kato K, Kawamura N, Kawanami M. The effects of collagen hydrogel implantation in buccal dehiscence defects in beagles. J Oral Tissue Eng 2007;5:87–95.

5

Primary Cell Culture from Human Dental Pulp

Futami Nagano-Takebe, Masaru Murata, Denis Selimovic, Kazuhiko Endo

The dental pulp is vascular connective tissue and is surrounded by hard tissue. The dental pulp has specific functions, such as repairing and forming dentin, providing nutrition for cellular elements, and imparting sensory feedback. This multifunctional tissue is composed of fibrils (mainly collagen), cells (such as fibroblasts, odontoblasts, and mesenchymal stem cells), matrix materials such as proteoglycans and fibronectins, blood vessels, and nerve tissue.[1,2]

Numerous publications have reported on stem cells, one of the key factors in tissue regeneration. Stem cells have the ability to proliferate and differentiate and can be isolated from a variety of tissues, such as bone marrow, skin, muscle, and adipose tissue. Recently, it has been reported that there are stem cells within human teeth, specifically in the dental pulp tissue and in the periodontal ligament. Gronthos et al[3] demonstrated that postnatal dental pulp contains cells that are highly proliferative and capable of regenerating tissue; these cells can therefore be defined as stem cells. These cells have been named *dental pulp stem cells* (DPSCs). Dental pulp tissue is easily obtained, for example, from sound teeth extracted for orthodontic treatment or from extracted healthy third molars. Compared with bone marrow stem cells, DPSCs have a stronger odontogenic capability and certainly generate dental tissues.[4] DPSCs are expected to serve as a stimulus for bone formation[5] and as a material to regenerate tissues in dentistry,[6–9] including nerve tissue.[10]

The scientific community has high expectations regarding the application of DPSCs to biomaterials, not only as a source but also as a substrate for cell differentiation and proliferation. Soria et al[11] reported that biomaterials covered with dental pulp cells acted as a scaffold, offering neurotrophic support for subsequent differentiation of neural stem cells. In addition, Van Wyk et al[12] demonstrated that cultured pulp fibroblasts showed strong sensitivity to toxic substances. These cells could, therefore, serve as a sensitive indicator of cytotoxicity.

Culturing of dental pulp–derived cells is commonplace in many laboratories. Some reports observe that the culture medium itself and the added reagents can influence the proliferation of human dental pulp cells.[13,14] The following is the procedure for basic culturing of primary human dental pulp cells.

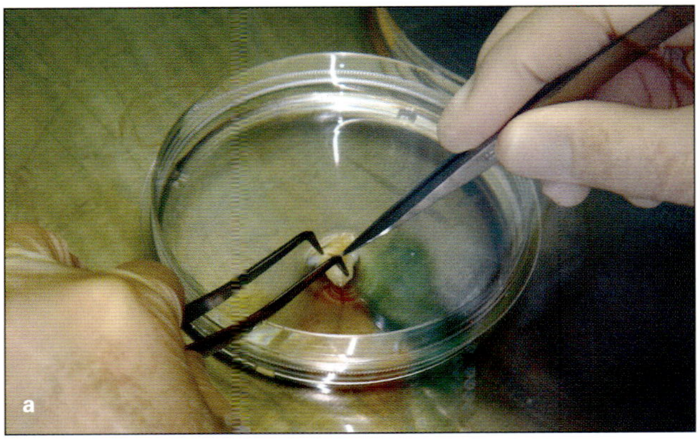

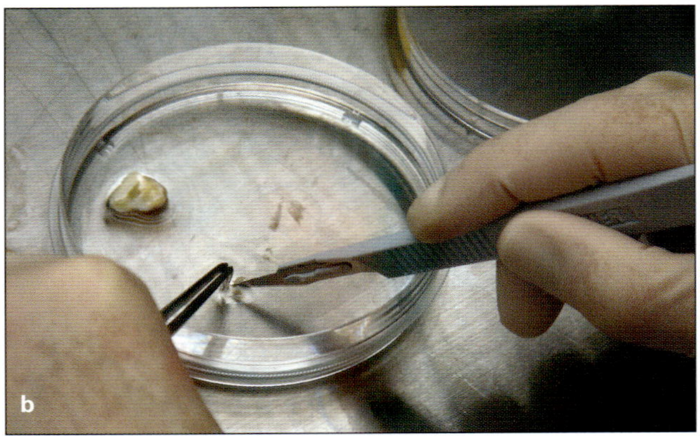

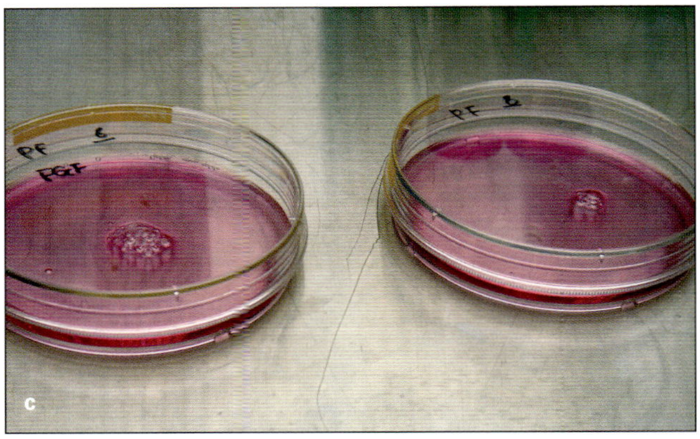

Fig 5-1 *(a to c)* The procedure for dental pulp extraction and placement in culture dishes.

Technical Procedure

Equipment and materials

Facilities and equipment required

1. Clean bench
2. Suction pump
3. Incubator
4. Inverted microscope
5. Pipettes and pipetter
6. Scalpels (no. 11, no. 15)
7. Plastic petri dishes (10 cm)
8. Pasteur pipettes
9. Sterile plastic tubes (50 mm)
10. Tweezers

Materials

1. Extracted human dental pulp tissue
2. Phosphate-buffered saline (PBS) without calcium or magnesium
3. Dulbecco's modified Eagle's medium (DMEM)
4. Penicillin (stock solution at 10,000 units/mL) and streptomycin (stock solution at 10 mg/mL)
5. Amphotericin B (stock solution at 250 µg/mL)
6. Fetal bovine serum (FBS)

Methods

Pulp extraction

The extracted tooth is kept in a plastic tube with sterile PBS that contains penicillin (100 units/mL) and streptomycin (0.1 mg/mL). The tooth is then washed several times with PBS to remove any attached blood. To obtain pulp from an extracted tooth, three different methods are used as follows:

1. A dental turbine is used with a diamond bur to cut the tooth vertical to the tooth axis at the cementoenamel junction. The pulp is extracted with a barbed broach or endodontic file.
2. The tooth is cut parallel to the tooth axis with a low-speed diamond saw (Isomet, Buehler) and the pulp extracted with tweezers.
3. The tooth is crushed (Dentmill, Tokyo Iken) with frozen cubes of PBS containing antimicrobial agents, and the pulp collected from the crushed tooth.

It is recommended that all procedures be performed on a clean bench. The extracted pulp is kept in the PBS containing an antibacterial agent or in DMEM containing 10% FBS, penicillin (100 units/mL), streptomycin (0.1 mg/mL), and amphotericin B (2.5 µg/mL).

Culturing pulp

Figure 5-1 shows the procedure for culturing pulp tissue. The extracted pulp is placed on a 10-cm dish. The tissue is cut into 2 × 2–mm pieces using sterile tweezers and scalpels. The pieces should then be washed several times in PBS containing antimicrobial agents; two or three pieces of pulp tissue are then placed in a new dish. A plastic dish that is coated

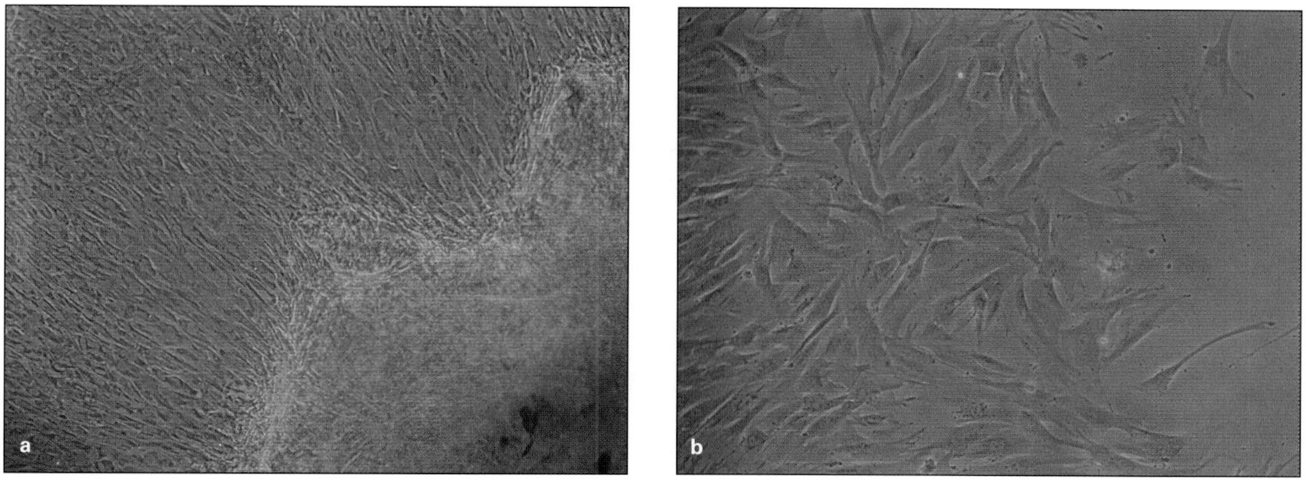

Fig 5-2 *(a, b)* The primary human dental pulp cells cultured from extracted dental pulp.

with collagen is most suitable for primary cell culture. Next, 5 mL of DMEM with the aforementioned agents is added gently to the dish.

To facilitate cell adhesion, the tissue should not float; rather, the pieces should attach to the bottom of the dish. The dish is placed into an incubator (5% carbon dioxide, 37°C). Oscillation of the dish should be avoided to prevent detachment of the tissue from the bottom of the dish.

The dish should be left undisturbed for 2 weeks. After 2 weeks, another 5 mL of DMEM can be added, gently pipetting down the side of the dish to avoid moving the tissue. After another 2 weeks, the cells should be attached firmly to the dish. Figure 5-2 shows primary human pulp cells that proliferated from the tissue. Fibroblasts are predominant in the culture dish. When the cells are attached firmly to the bottom of the dish, the medium should be changed every 3 days. It will take approximately 1 to 2 months for primary pulp cells obtained from an adult in his or her early 20s to reach 80% confluence on a dish. Pulp cells from an older adult will take longer to grow than those from a young adult or child. Pulp harvested from an older person will also include more fibrils and fewer cells than will pulp obtained from a young adult. The number of cells that will be acquired for culturing would therefore be fewer than in young pulp. In such cases, it can be useful to incubate pulp tissue with collagenase to help decompose the collagen fibrils in the pulp tissue.

Conclusions

Establishing cultures of human pulp–derived cells is not difficult as long as the experimental environment is kept sterile and antimicrobial agents are used immediately after extraction of the tooth. The oral cavity is a hotbed of bacteria, so protection of the tissue and cells from bacterial contamination is vital for the successful establishment of human pulp–derived cells.

References

1. Hu JW. Tooth pulp. In: Miles TS, Nauntofte B, Svensson P (eds). Clinical Oral Physiology. Copenhagen: Quintessence, 2004:141–164.
2. Avery JK, Chiego DJ Jr. Dental pulp. In: Avery JK, Chiege DJ Jr (eds). Essentials of Oral Histology and Embryology: A Clinical Approach, ed 3. St Louis: Mosby, 2006:121–136.
3. Gronthos S, Mankani M, Brahim J, Robey P, Shi S. Postnatal human dental pulp stem cells (DPSCs) in vitro and in vivo. Proc Natl Acad Sci U S A 2000;97:13625–13630.
4. Yu J, Wang Y, Deng Z, et al. Odontogenic capability: Bone marrow stromal stem cells versus dental pulp stem cells. Biol Cell 2007;99:465–474.
5. Ikeda H, Sumita Y, Ikeda M, et al. Engineering bone formation from human dental pulp- and periodontal ligament-derived cells. Ann Biomed Eng 2011;39:26–34.
6. Mooney DJ, Powell C, Piana J, Rutherford B. Engineering dental pulp-like tissue in vitro. Biotechnol Prog 1996;12:865–868.
7. Graziano A, d'Aquino R, Laino G, Papaccio G. Dental pulp stem cells: A promising tool for bone regeneration. Stem Cell Rev 2008;4:21–26.
8. Telles PD, Machado MA, Sakai VT, Nör JE. Pulp tissue from primary teeth: New source of stem cells. J Appl Oral Sci 2011;19:189–194.
9. Casagrande L, Cordeiro MM, Nör SA, Nör JE. Dental pulp stem cells in regenerative dentistry. Odontology 2011;99:1–7.
10. Nourbakhsh N, Soleimani M, Taghipour Z, et al. Induced in vitro differentiation of neural-like cells from human exfoliated deciduous teeth-derived stem cells. Int J Dev Biol 2011;55:189–195.
11. Soria JM, Sancho-Tello M, Esparza MA, et al. Biomaterials coated by dental pulp cells as substrate for neural stem cell differentiation. J Biomed Mater Res A 2011;97:85–92.
12. Van Wyk CW, Oliver A, Maritz JS. Cultured pulp fibroblasts: Are they suitable for in vitro cytotoxicity testing? J Oral Pathol Med 2001;30:168–177.
13. Pissiotis E, Spangberg L. The importance of the culture medium on human dental pulp cell attachment. Arch Oral Biol 1993; 38:641–647.
14. Cortes O, Garcia C, Perez L, Boj J, Alcaina A. Pulp cell cultures obtained with two different methods for in vitro cytotoxicity tests. Eur Arch Paediatr Dent 2006;7:95–99.

6

Detection of BMP-2 in Human Dental Pulp

Katsutoshi Ito, Toshiya Arakawa, Masaru Murata, Kaoru Kusano, Junichi Tazaki, Md Arafat Kabir, Taishin Takuma

The dental pulp plays two important roles: *(1)* formation and maintenance of dentin and *(2)* sensing any irritation that teeth receive. It is well known that the pulp chamber and root canal of immature permanent teeth are larger and wider than those of mature teeth (Fig 6-1). They become narrow after reparative dentin (secondary dentin and tertiary dentin) is formed by dental pulp tissue when root formation is complete. Secondary dentin grows on the inner surface of the pulp chamber with age and as a result of occlusal forces (Fig 6-2); tertiary dentin, which functions like a dentin "bridge," is formed by external stimulation such as dental caries (Fig 6-3). Bone morphogenetic proteins (BMPs), which belong to the transforming growth factor-ß superfamily, are multifunctional growth factors related to bone formation and embryogenesis. It is well known that BMPs are involved in dentin formation in dental pulp as strong influences on hard tissue morphogenesis.

Studies have demonstrated that bone and dentin can be formed in ectopic transplantation using pulp from dog and rabbit teeth and that dentin with dentinal tubules can be formed in autogenous transplantation using pulp from rat teeth,[1,2] although BMP-2 was originally detected in bone.[3] Thus, there is a possibility that BMP-2 exists in dental pulp.

Human BMP-2 and BMP-4 were cloned in 1988, and expression of the mRNA of BMP-2, BMP-4, and BMP-6 was identified in primary culture cells of human dental pulp.[4] The expression of mRNA in adult human dental pulp tissue was examined by reverse-transcription polymerase chain reaction (RT-PCR) for detection of BMP-2, BMP-4, and osteogenic protein-1 (BMP-7) in 1996.[5] However, the detection levels of BMPs as protein were unclear.

Recombinant human BMP-2 is now available for orthopedic and dental use in the United States; the Food and Drug Administration cleared the clinical application of BMP-2 in 2002. Implantation of BMP-2 induces new bone formation; thus, it can be used for bony defects. BMP-2 is the strongest of the BMPs, involving not only the formation of bone but also other hard tissues such as reparative dentin. In the present study, the expression of proteins of BMP-2 in human dental pulp was determined, and the presence of BMP-2 in dental pulp was investigated.

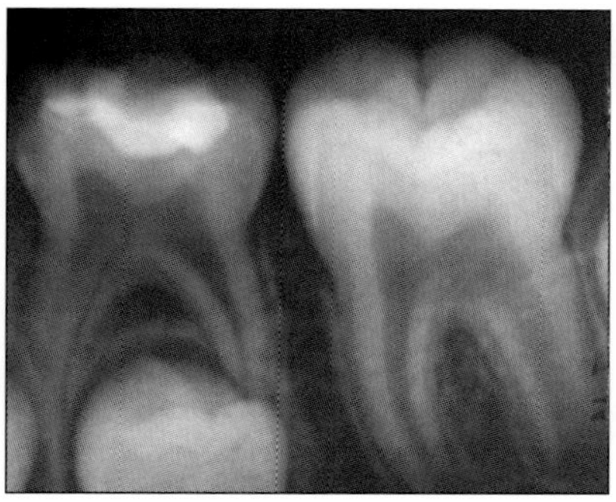

Fig 6-1 Immature permanent mandibular left first molar. The pulp chamber and root canals are large and wide.

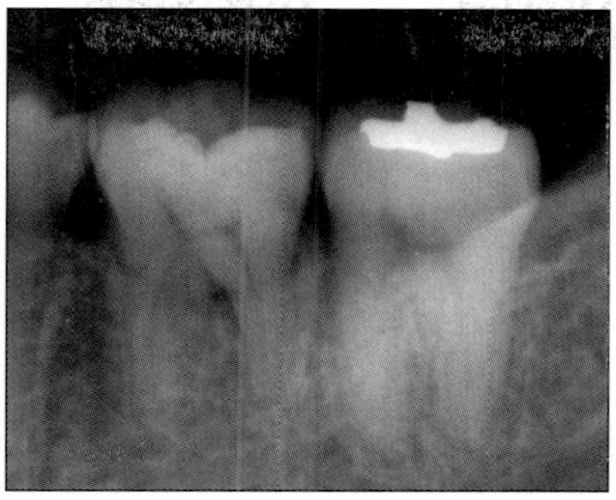

Fig 6-2 Permanent mandibular left first molar. Secondary dentin is formed on the inner surface of the pulp chamber.

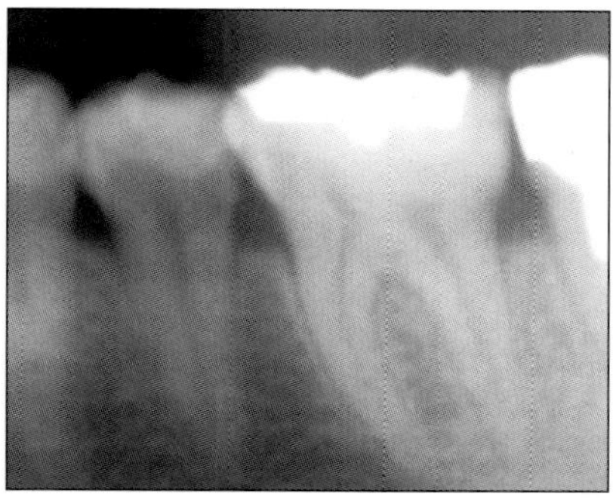

Fig 6-3 Permanent mandibular left first molar. Tertiary dentin has formed on the inner surface of the pulp chamber.

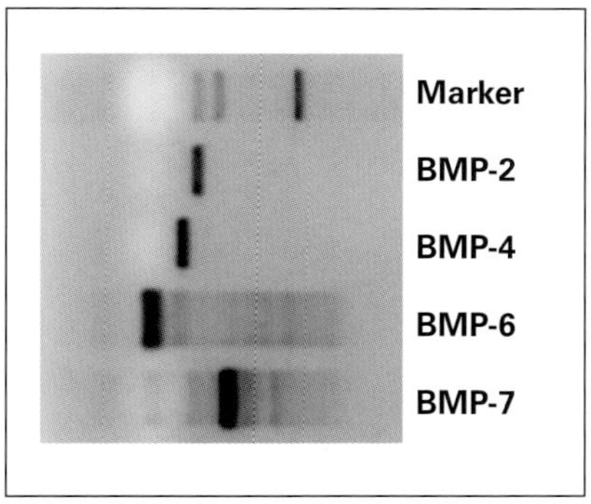

Fig 6-4 Expression of mRNA of BMPs in human dental pulp tissue.

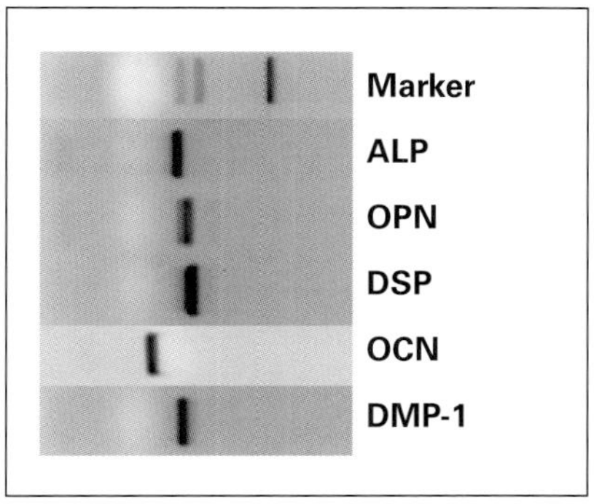

Fig 6-5 Expression of mRNA of hard tissue–related factors in human dental pulp tissue.

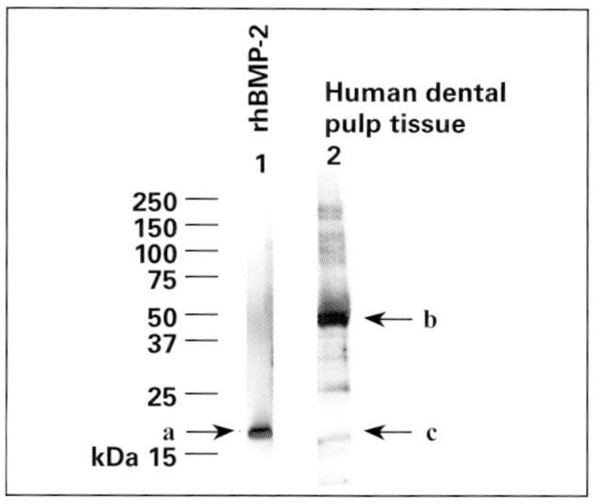

Fig 6-6 Detection of BMP-2 in human dental pulp by Western blot analysis.

Methods

Human dental pulp tissue was obtained from normal and caries superficialis third molars of adult patients (20 to 30 years old) that had been extracted for valid clinical reasons. Total RNA was isolated from the dental pulp tissue using TRIzol reagent (Invitrogen, Life Technologies). Next, cDNA was constructed from 1 μg of the total RNA via RT using SuperScript III (Invitrogen). PCR was performed using Plutinum Taq (Invitrogen) and KOD Plus (Toyobo). The lysates of the dental pulp tissues and cells were electrophoresed in sodium dodecyl sulfate polyacrylamide gel electrophoresis (SDS-PAGE). Western blot analysis was performed using mouse monoclonal anti-human BMP-2 antibodies (R&D Systems). After the membrane was treated with goat anti-mouse gamma G immunoglobulin antibody (Amersham, Invitrogen), the bands were detected using ECL Plus (Amersham, Invitrogen).

Results

PCR analysis indicated that BMP-2, BMP-4, BMP-6, BMP-7, alkaline phosphatase (ALP), osteopontin (OPN), dentin sialoprotein (DSP), osteocalcin (OCN), and dentin matrix acidic phosphoprotein 1 (DMP-1) were expressed in human dental pulp tissue (Figs 6-4 and 6-5).

The presence of mature recombinant human BMP-2 was demonstrated by a major band at 16 kDa (Fig 6-6, lane 1, *arrow a*) in a reduced condition by Western blot analysis with dental pulp tissue. BMP-2 in human dental pulp was additionally demonstrated by a major band at 50 kDa (Fig 6-6, lane 2, *arrow b*) and by a minor band at 16 kDa (Fig 6-6, lane 2, *arrow c*) in a reduced condition.

Discussion

It is thought that formation of reparative dentin is related to age, dental caries, crown restoration, and attrition.[6] It has been reported that the mRNA of BMP-2 and BMP-4 was expressed ahead of ALP in cultured dental pulp cells and then the cells were calcified. The present study confirmed the presence of mRNA of BMPs and hard tissue–related factors in human dental pulp. These results suggest that the osteogenic activity of dental pulp tissue is stimulated by BMPs and their related factors. Previous studies identified mRNA expression of BMPs and hard tissue–related factors; however, the proteins of these factors were not identified clearly in human dental pulp. BMPs are produced as a 50-kDa precursor and migrate at 16 kDa as a mature protein by processing in a reduced condition.[7] In this study (see Fig 6-6), the protein of BMP in dental pulp tissue was analyzed by Western blot analysis, and a major band at 50 kDa and a minor band at 16 kDa were detected in reduced conditions.[8] Thus, BMP-2 in dental pulp exists as a high molecular weight precursor, and dental pulp tissue might be used as an osteoinductive material if its precursor could be intentionally matured at an accelerated pace.

Conclusion

The following can be concluded from this study:

1. mRNAs of BMP-2, BMP-4, BMP-6, BMP-7, ALP, OPN, DSP, OCN, and DMP-1 were expressed in human dental pulp tissues.
2. BMP-2 in human dental pulp tissue existed as a 50-kDa precursor form in reduced condition.

These results indicate that human dental pulp might contribute to bone formation as an osteoinductive tissue that includes stem cells.

References

1. Yamamura T, Shimono M, Koike H, et al. Differentiation and induction of undifferentiated mesenchymal cells in tooth and periodontal tissue during wound healing and regeneration. Bull Tokyo Dent Coll 1980;21:181–221
2. Inoue T, Tanaka Y, Shimono M, Yamamura T. Osteogenic activity of transplanted dental pulp. Jpn J Oral Biol 1984;26:1344–1346.
3. Urist MR. Bone: Formation by autoinduction. Science 1965;150: 893–899.
4. Takeda K, Oida S, Goseki M, et al. Expression of bone morphogenetic protein genes in the human dental pulp cells. Bone 1994; 15:467–470.
5. Gu K, Smoke RH, Rutherford RB. Expression of genes for bone morphogenetic proteins and receptors in human dental pulp. Arch Oral Biol 1996;41:919–923.
6. Yaegashi T, Satoh T, Yasuge T, et al. Expression of genes in relation to calcification of dental pulp cell. Jpn J Conserv Dent 2000;43:46.
7. Israel DI, Nove J, Kerns KM, Moutsatsos IK, Kaufman RJ. Expression and characterization of bone morphogenetic protein-2 in Chinese hamster ovary cells. Growth Factors 1992; 7:139–150.
8. Ito K, Arakawa T, Murata M, Takuma T, Arisue M. Expression of bone morphogenetic proteins (BMPs) in human dental pulp. J Hard Tissue Biol 2007;16:199–204.

7

Detection of Bacteria in Human Tooth–Derived Biomaterials

Mari Fujita, Osamu Uehara, Hiroshi Miyakawa, Sumiyoshi Naito, Md Arafat Kabir, Masaru Murata, Futoshi Nakazawa

In recent years, autogenous tooth tissue has been developed as a novel bone grafting material.[1–3] For this application, an extracted tooth stored in cell-freezing medium is crushed, demineralized, and treated with antibacterial agents. Then the crushed tooth is lyophilized and used as demineralized dentin matrix (DDM). Because the extracted tooth is not sterilized during this process, DDM granules may be contaminated with oral bacteria.[4] Thus, it is very important to determine whether oral bacteria are present in these biomaterials to reduce the risk of infection. However, it is well known that almost all bacteria in the human oral cavity are anaerobic, and culture of these bacteria should be done under strict anaerobic conditions.[5] Therefore, the present study examined bacterial contamination of stored teeth and prepared DDM granules through the use of culture techniques under strict anaerobic conditions.

Bacterial Culture Tests

To assay viable bacteria in the cell-freezing medium (Bambanker, LYMPHOTEC) that was used to store an extracted tooth (Fig 7-1), the medium was inoculated with brain-heart infusion broth (BHI broth, BD Diagnostic Systems) supplemented with 1.5% (by volume) agar, 5 mg/mL hemin, 4 mg/mL menadione, and 5% (by volume) defimbriated sheep blood (Nippon Biotest Lab) (BHI-HM blood agar) after a 10-fold serial dilution. This was incubated at 37°C under both aerobic and strict anaerobic conditions in an anaerobic chamber with an atmosphere of 80% nitrogen, 10% hydrogen, and 10% carbon dioxide. After 72 to 96 hours, the total number of colony-forming units (CFU) per milliliter was determined (bacterial culture test 1).

Many bacteria were detected in the cell-freezing medium: 2.2×10^5 CFU/mL in aerobic cultures and 3.5×10^5 CFU/mL in anaerobic cultures (Fig 7-2a). These results suggest that the autogenous tooth stored in the cell-freezing medium was possibly contaminated by oral bacteria.

To detect bacteria in the DDM granules, 25 mg of lyophilized DDM granules (0.5 to 1.0 mm) were homogenized with 1 mL of phosphate-buffered saline, and the suspension was inoculated in BHI-HM blood agar after a 10-fold serial dilution (bacterial culture test 2). Also, 25 mg of the lyophilized DDM granules were inoculated directly in 5 mL of BHI broth supplemented with hemin and menadione and incubated at 37°C under aerobic and anaerobic conditions. After 48 hours, the cultured medium was inoculated on BHI-HM blood agar after a 10-fold serial dilution (bacterial culture test 3). Finally, bacteria in the DDM granules (bacterial culture tests 2 and 3) were cultured and examined in the same manner as in bacterial culture test 1.

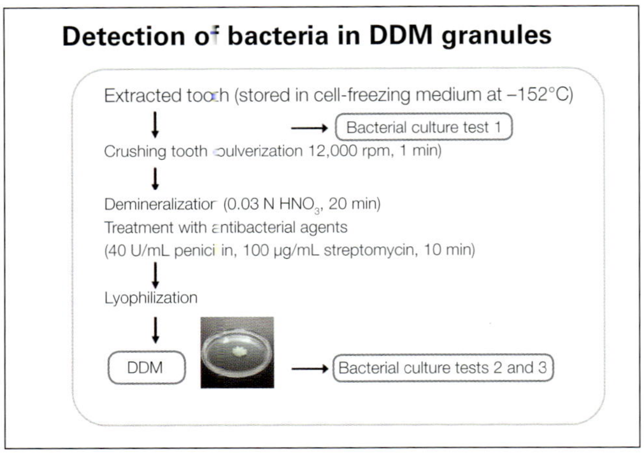

Fig 7-1 Procedures for preparation of DDM granules and bacterial culture tests. Bacterial counts were determined in the cell-freezing medium used to store the extracted tooth (bacterial culture test 1) and in the DDM granules (bacterial culture tests 2 and 3).

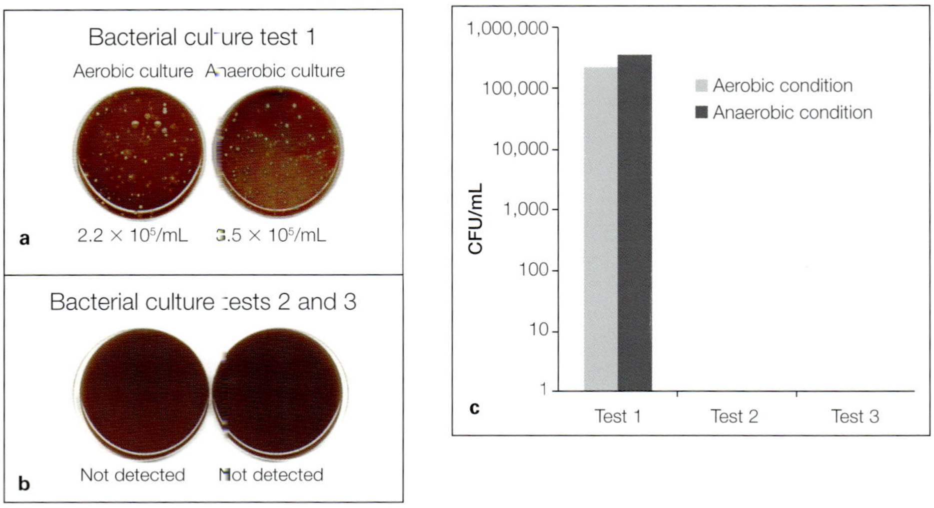

Fig 7-2 Results of bacterial culture tests. *(a,b)* BHI-HM blood agars cultured under aerobic *(left)* and anaerobic *(right)* conditions. *(c)* Total CFU/mL for all three tests.

Bacterial culture tests 2 and 3 indicated that no viable bacteria were detected in the DDM granules (Fig 7-2b). These results suggest that bacterial contamination of DDM granules was reduced by demineralization and treatment with antibacterial agents (Fig 7-2c).

Conclusion

This study demonstrated that viable bacteria were not detected in DDM granules, even though the stored tooth was contaminated with a great deal of oral bacteria. The result in the highly sensitive blood agar medium was comparable to a previous test culture (7 days in Thioglycollate medium with vitamin K and hemin).[3] These results suggest that the demineralization and/or antibacterial treatments might reduce bacterial contamination significantly. DDM granules from autogenous tooth material can be applied for bone grafts and used as a biomaterial, thus allowing improvement of bone induction while reducing the risk of infection.

References

1. Murata M, Akazawa T, Takahata M, et al. Bone induction of human tooth and bone crushed by newly developed automatic mill. J Ceram Soc Jpn 2010;118:434–437.
2. Murata M, Kawai T, Kawakami T, et al. Human acid-insoluble dentin with BMP-2 accelerates bone induction in subcutaneous and intramuscular tissues. J Ceram Soc Jpn 2010;118:438–441.
3. Tazaki J, Murata M, Yuasa T, et al. Autograft of human tooth and demineralized dentin matrices for bone augmentation. J Ceram Soc Jpn 2010;118:442–445.
4. Etcheson AW, Miley DD, Gillespie MJ. Osseous coagulum collected in bone traps: Potential for bacterial contamination and methods for decontamination. J Oral Implantol 2007;33:109–115.
5. Uematsu H, Hoshino E. Predominant obligate anaerobes in human periodontal pockets. J Periodontal Res 1992;27:15–19.
6. Ando N, Hoshino E, Sato M, et al. Culture conditions for efficient recovery of bacteria from infected dental root canals. Jpn J Oral Biol 1989; 31:603–608.

8

Subcutaneous Implantation of Demineralized Dentin Matrix

Jun Hino, Masaru Murata, Junichi Tazaki, Katsutoshi Ito, Yasuhito Minamida, Md Arafat Kabir, Izumi Asahina, Takanori Shibata

In 1965, bone morphogenetic protein was first discovered in bone matrix.[1] In 1967, the bone-inducing property of rabbit and rat dentin was discovered via implantation in intramuscular pockets.[2,3] Murata et al[4] confirmed the osteoinductive property of human demineralized dentin matrix (DDM) granules in the subcutaneous tissue of 4-week-old male athymic mice. This chapter demonstrates bone induction by subcutaneous implantation of human DDM in mice, as well as the difference in appearance in the giant cells in the organic DDM compared with those in inorganic material like hydroxyapatite.

Experimental Method

Experimental animals

All animal procedures were performed in accordance with the experimental guidelines for animals at the Health Sciences University of Hokkaido, and the protocol was approved by the Managements Committee of the Laboratory Animal Center at the Health Sciences University of Hokkaido. Four-week-old male athymic mice (weight of 30 g) were used in this study.

Conventional preparation of human DDM

First, human impacted mandibular teeth were extracted and preserved at –80°C. They were then crushed to a size between 400 and 800 µm. The material was washed for 90 minutes in sodium chloride solution (pH 7.4), defatted for 180 minutes in a 1:1 mixture of chloroform and methanol, and washed for 120 minutes in 100% methanol. The material was then decalcified for 15 hours in hydrochloric acid (pH 2.0), washed for 120 minutes in Tris–hydrochloric acid (pH 7.4), and freeze-dried for 12 hours.

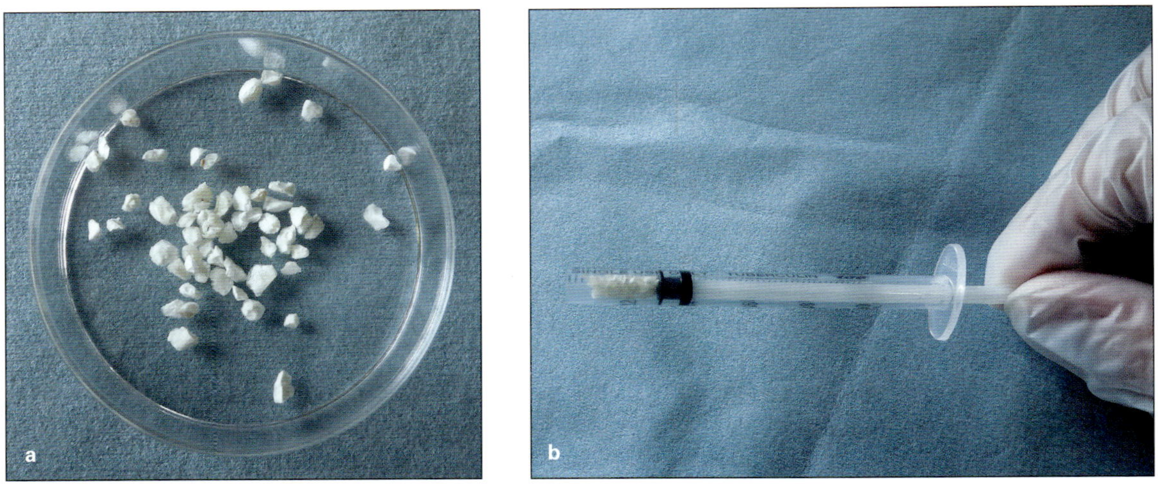

Fig 8-1 *(a)* Freeze-dried human DDM. *(b)* Human DDM in a syringe.

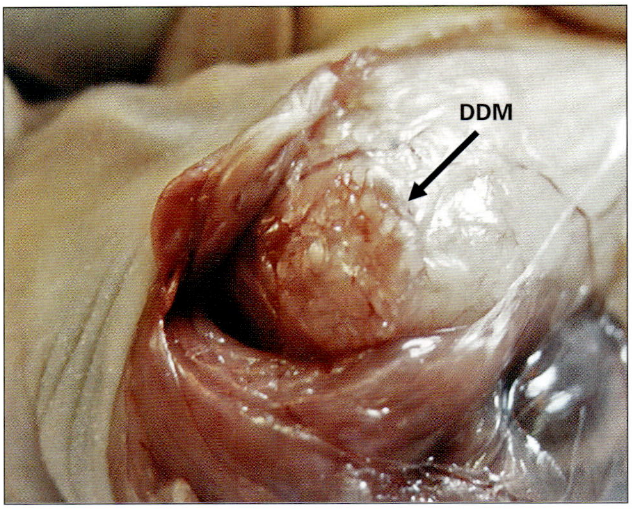

Fig 8-2 Exposure of implanted DDM in subcutaneous tissue after 4 weeks.

Subcutaneous implantation

For implantation into mice, the human DDM material was inserted into a syringe (Fig 8-1), soaked in 100 mL of phosphate-buffered saline, and preserved at –80°C. Subcutaneous implantation of the DDM into the athymic mice was performed under general anesthesia.

Histologic examination

Four weeks after subcutaneous implantation, all mice were killed by ether overdose, and each implanted specimen of DDM was retrieved as a mass (Fig 8-2). All samples were fixed in neutral buffered 10% formalin and embedded in paraffin. Four-micrometer sections were cut and stained with hematoxylin-eosin (HE) for light microscopic observation.

Result

DDM induced growth of both bone and cartilage. New bone with osteoblast lining was found on the surface of the DDM (Fig 8-3). Cartilage was induced between DDM particles (Fig 8-4). Giant cells appeared, and cellular absorption was observed locally (Fig 8-5).

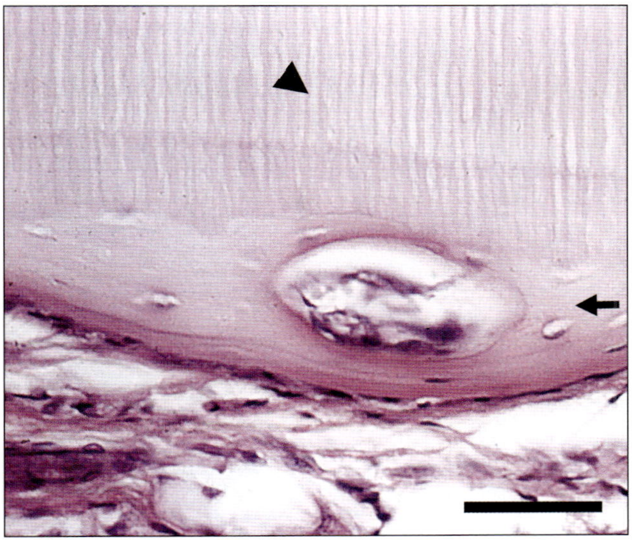

Fig 8-3 Induced bone *(arrow)* on the DDM surface *(arrowhead)*, with osteoblast lining. Note the relationship in vertical position between new bone and arrangement of dentinal tube spaces (HE; bar = 20 µm).

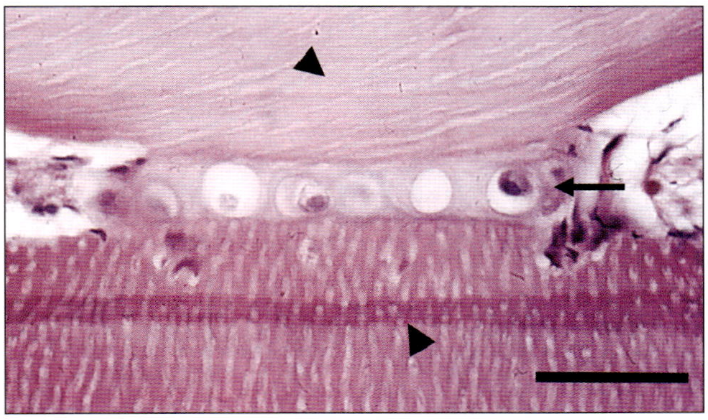

Fig 8-4 Induced cartilage *(arrow)* between DDM particles *(arrowheads)* (HE; bar = 20 µm).

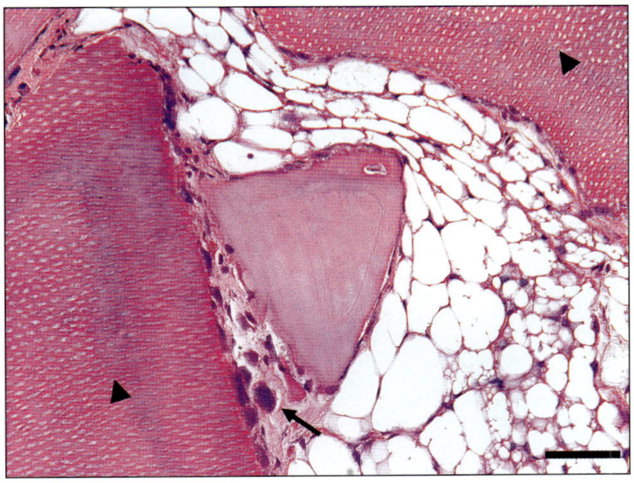

Fig 8-5 A few giant cells *(arrow)* were found on the surface layer of the DDM particles *(arrowheads)* (HE; bar = 20 µm).

Table 8-1 Morphometry of implanted tissue after 4 weeks (n = 3)

Tissue	Area % (mean ± SD)
Bone	0.9 ± 0.1
Cartilage	0.4 ± 0.2
Bone marrow	0.4 ± 0.1
DDM	74.7 ± 4.9
Mesenchymal tissue	23.6 ± 5.0

SD = standard deviation.

Morphometric analysis revealed percentages of induced bone, cartilage, and bone marrow of 0.9% ± 0.1%, 0.4% ± 0.2%, and 0.4% ± 0.1%, respectively. The average percentage of DDM was 74.7% ± 4.9% (Table 8-1).

Discussion

The demineralization of bone and dentin increases their osteoinductivity and decreases their antigenecity.[5] Many researchers have reported the phenomenon of bone induction by DDM.[2,3,6–8] In this study, human DDM induced the growth of bone and cartilage. However, the morphometric analysis indicated that bone-inducing properties of human DDM were weak.

The DDM occupied, on average, 74.7% of the volume of the total tissues. DDM is a highly insoluble type I collagenous matrix, and degradation of DDM is caused by tissue collagenase. The authors also performed subcutaneous implantation of hydroxyapatite blocks (APACERAM-AX, HOYA; 3 mm^3) in the same procedure. Histologic examination showed that giant cells were fairly common in these tissues (Fig 8-6, Table 8-2); in contrast, giant cells in the implanted DDM tissues appeared locally and were less frequent.

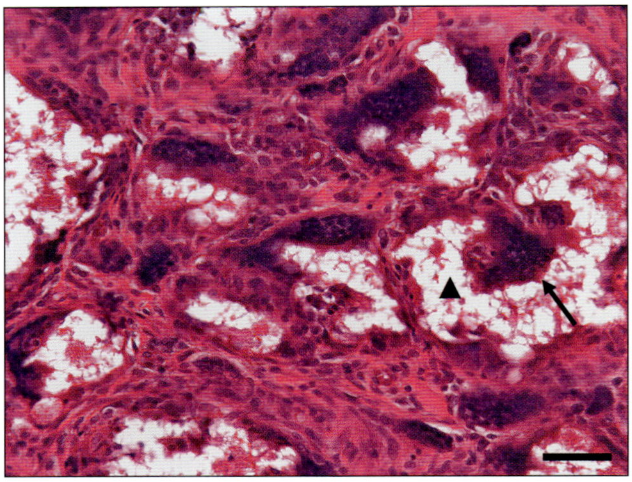

Fig 8-6 Histologic appearance after 4 weeks of subcutaneous implantation of hydroxyapatite. Many giant cells *(arrow)* were found on the surface of hydroxyapatite *(arrowhead)* (HE; bar = 20 µm).

Table 8-2	**Mean no. of giant cells in implanted tissue after 4 weeks**
Tissue	**No. of cells (± SD)**
DDM	2.7 ± 1.5
Hydroxyapatite	11.3 ± 2.1

Values are per 250 × 250 µm.
n = 3, $P < .05$ (Student *t* test).

Conclusion

These results indicate that particles of DDM derived from extracted human teeth are collagenous matrices with chondro-osteoinductive potential.

References

1. Urist MR. Bone: Formation by autoinduction. Science 1965;150: 893–899.
2. Yeomans JD, Urist MR. Bone induction by decalcified dentine implanted into oral, osseous and muscle tissue. Arch Oral Biol 1967;12:999–1008.
3. Bang G, Urist MR. Bone induction in excavation chambers in matrix of decalcified dentin. Arch Surg 1967;94:781–789.
4. Murata M, Sato D, Akazawa T, Taira T, Sasaki T, Arisue M. Bone and cartilage induction in nude mice by human demineralized dentin matrix. J Hard Tissue Biol 2003;11:110–114.
5. Reddi AH. Bone matrix in the solid state: Geometric influence on differentiation of fibroblasts. Adv Biol Med Phys 1974; 15:1-18.
6. Huggins C, Wiseman S, Reddi AH. Transformation of fibroblasts by allogeneic and xenogeneic transplants of demineralized tooth and bone. J Exp Med 1970;132:1250–1258.
7. Butler WT, Mikulski A, Urist MR, Bridges G, Uyeno S. Noncollagenous proteins of a rat dentin matrix possessing bone morphogenetic activity. J Dent Res 1977;56:228–232.
8. Bessho K, Tanaka N, Matsumoto J, Tagawa T, Murata M. Human dentin-matrix-derived bone morphogenetic protein. J Dent Res 1991;70:171–175.

9

Surface Design and Functional Control of Demineralized Dentin Matrix

Toshiyuki Akazawa, Masaru Murata, Jun Hino, Katsuo Nakamura, Masahiko Kikuchi, Masaharu Mitsugi, In-Woong Um

In conjunction with increases in aging populations, cases of periodontal disease and osteoporosis have been on the rise. Thus, safe and easy treatments are required. Materials originating from living tissues feature their original morphology, a reasonable surface structure, and a chemical nature (acidic-basic strength) affected by small amounts of metal ions in a living environment. Biomimetic organic and inorganic materials are functional composites that are effective in maintaining an optimal environment for cells or biopolymers. However, with respect to bone-regenerative therapy, researchers have continued to focus on the development and application of biomimetic biomaterials because they are not only degradable and absorbable in vivo but also can accelerate the metabolism of living hard tissues.[1]

The human tooth comprises mostly enamel in the surface layer, dentin in the second layer, and dental pulp inside. Dentin is a composite of apatite and collagen. In dentin, microscopic amounts of physiologically active substances (eg, bone morphogenetic proteins [BMPs]) and calcification-accelerating substances are adsorbed on collagen.[2]

In 2004, because of the need to safely recycle and reuse autologous teeth (extracted teeth) from patients, the authors created a human tooth bank at the Health Sciences University of Hokkaido to contribute to regenerative therapy, such as reconstruction of the alveolar process and bone to support natural teeth. Depending on the location and volume of material obtained and required, the extracted teeth were recycled as various granules, pulverized for use in later bone regenerative therapy in each patient.[3] The typical process of pulverizing extracted teeth was carried out by grinding them with a stainless metal/agate mortar and pestle for about 30 minutes, together with liquid nitrogen, to prevent the denaturation of proteins or other physiologically active substances. However, it is very difficult to manually control the particle size and distribution of the granules with this technique.

It was previously demonstrated that demineralized dentin matrix (DDM) granules, including small patches of cementum derived from extracted teeth, induced bone and cartilage growth independently in the subcutaneous tissues of nude mice.[4] Since DDM granules are osteoinductive and made up of insoluble collagen matrix, they should serve as effective carriers of bone growth factors for bone regenerative therapy. However, the ability of the ground granules to dissolve and the hydroxyapatite (HA) content of DDM might influence osteoinduction of DDM granules, because HA crystals inhibit BMP release in vivo.

To apply recycled extracted teeth for therapy in the orofacial region, it is important to tailor the granules to the patient's need, which can be done with a small cooling-pulverizing apparatus within a very short time, and to demineralize them as soon as possible. This chapter introduces research and development of a small cooling-pulverizing apparatus for extracted teeth, discusses the granules that are created with the apparatus, and de-

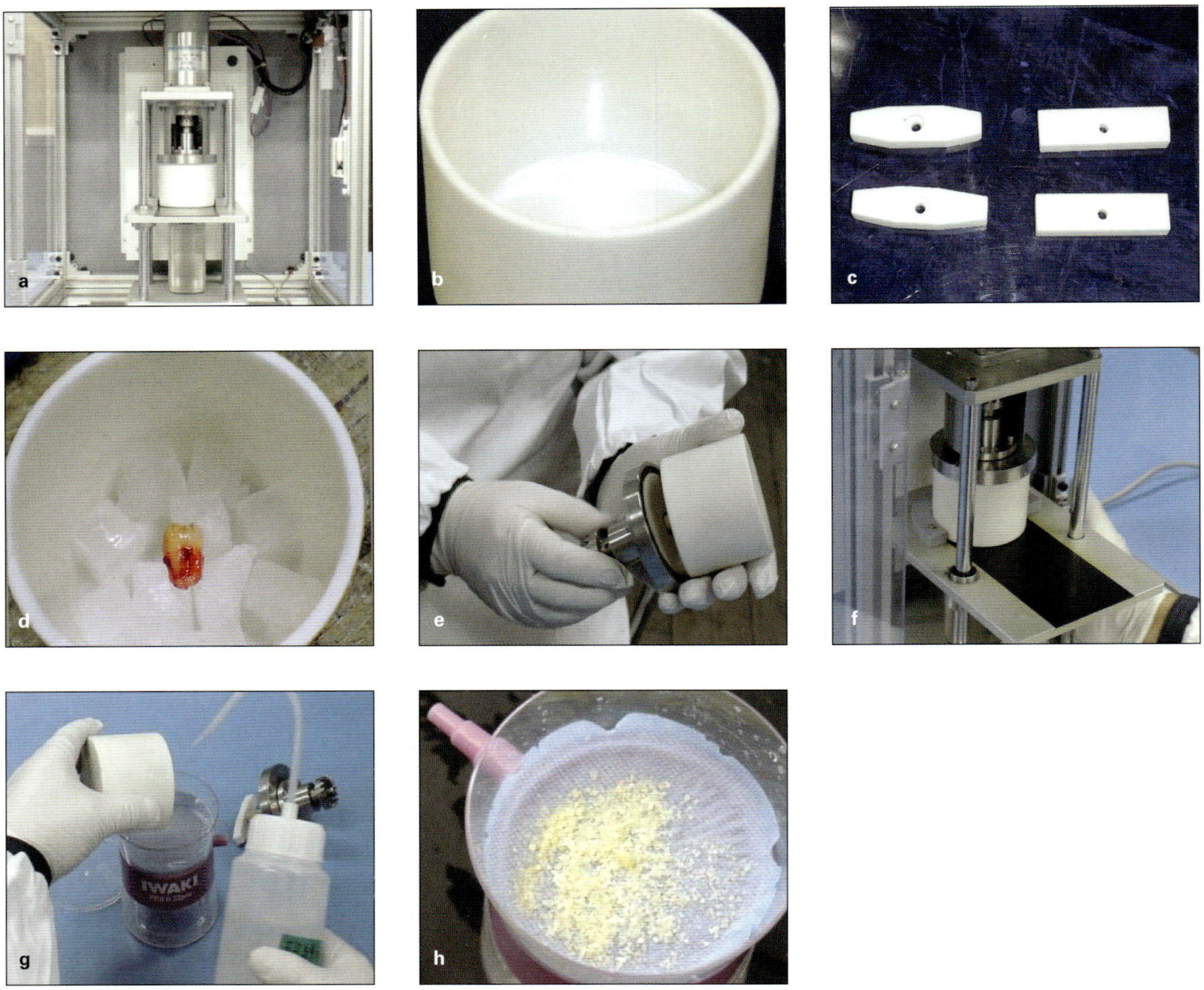

Fig 9-1 *(a)* Pulverizing apparatus with cooling mechanism and high rotational speed for reuse of human teeth. With the apparatus, extracted human teeth are pulverized with saline ice for 1 minute at 12,000 rpm with a zirconia blade in a zirconia vessel. *(b)* The zirconia vessel. *(c)* Zirconia rotational blades. *(d)* Extracted human tooth and 20 cubes of saline ice. *(e)* Capping of the operculum with zirconia rotational blade attached. *(f)* The zirconia vessel is carefully positioned inside the apparatus, and the tooth is pulverized by rotation of the zirconia blade. *(g)* Collection of the sample slurry. *(h)* Aspiration, filtration, and washing of the pulverized granules.

scribes the excellent surface characteristics and functions of these biomimetic materials modified by both the demineralization and specific precipitation processes.

Cooling-Pulverizing Technique for Reuse of Human Teeth

Zirconia ceramic vessels and rotational blades with high mechanical strength and excellent durability in acid were fabricated by the slip casting method to be used as pulverizing units for extracted teeth.[5] The zirconia slurry was milled with a zirconia ball for 24 hours, evacuated, and cast onto some gypsum plates. The detached and dried zirconia vessels (cylindric in shape) and rotational blades (rectangle or rhombus shape) were sintered at 1,673 to 1,773 K for 2 hours in air. Zirconia ceramics sintered at 1,673 K exhibit 21% calcination shrinkage, 6.05 cm^3/g bulk density, 99% relative density, and 400 MPa bending strength; all of these values are sufficient for pulverizing and processing extracted teeth.

After a zirconia vessel and a zirconia rotational blade were attached to a small pulverizing apparatus, extracted human

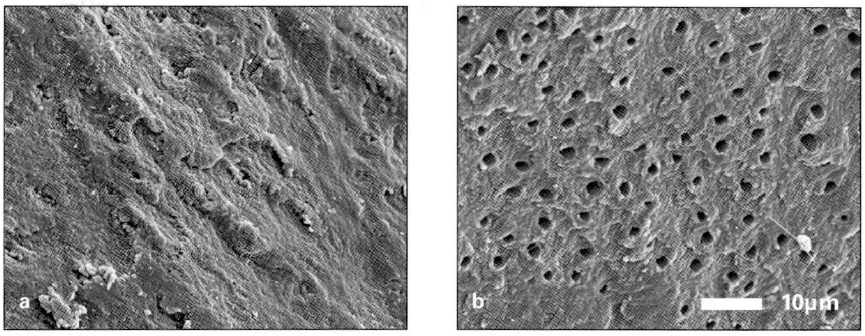

Fig 9-2 SEM images of human tooth granules after pulverization with saline ice for 1 minute under 12,000 rpm with a zirconia blade in a zirconia vessel. *(a)* Microstructure of the pulverized granules from an extracted tooth. *(b)* Microstructure of the pulverized granules of dentin after exclusion of the enamel.

teeth were pulverized with saline ice for 0.5 to 2 minutes at 9,000 to 12,000 rpm to prevent thermal denaturation of any physiologically active substances and calcification-accelerating substances.[6] Figures 9-1a to 9-1c show the pulverizing apparatus, which incorporates a cooling mechanism and high rotational speeds. An extracted human tooth and 20 pieces of saline ice were loaded into the zirconia vessel (Fig 9-1d). The vessel was capped by an operculum with the blade attached to it and set onto the pulverizing apparatus (Fig 9-1e). The position of the vessel was carefully controlled before rotating the blade at 12,000 rpm for 1 minute to pulverize the extracted tooth (Figs 9-1f). During the pulverization, some saline ice remained in the vessel so that the temperature inside the vessel was kept below 273 K. After the vessel was removed from the apparatus and the operculum was opened, the sample slurry was collected on a filter paper (Fig 9-1g). Finally, it was filtrated by aspiration and washed with large amounts of saline solution (Fig 9-1h).

The pulverized granules exhibited ideal particle sizes (0.5 to 2 mm) for regeneration of alveolar bone. Scanning electron microscopic (SEM) photographs of the granules were taken to investigate the morphology and microstructure of the granules. Figure 9-2 shows SEM photographs of human teeth pulverized together with saline ice. After the enamel portion of the human tooth was excluded, many dentinal tubules, 1 to 2 mm in size, were clearly observed in the granules.

The ratio of calcium to phosphate ions (Ca/P) was determined by electron probe microanalysis. The Ca/P ratios of the granules were 1.60 to 1.66, which are close to the stoichiometric value of 1.67 for standard HA. The other constituents were analyzed using inductively coupled plasma. Small amounts of sodium and magnesium ions, present in less than 1% of the weight, were detected. In analyses of all the pulverized granules, zirconium was not detected, suggesting that the abrasive powder of zirconia was not incorporated from the zirconia ceramic during pulverizing and processing.[1]

Effects of Acid Dissolution on DDM Granules

The pulverized granules were dissolved under 500 rpm at room temperature and pH 1 for 3 hours in 0.3% to 2.0% nitric acid or hydrochloric acid aqueous solutions to obtain DDM granules. To control the velocity of the release of bone growth factors from dentin, the acid treatment conditions, such as concentration of the aqueous solutions, holding time, and liquid temperature, were investigated for their efficacy in the demineralization process, ie, excluding the mineral components of enamel and dentin from human teeth.

The crystalline phase of the samples was identified by micro–x-ray diffraction using K-α1 radiation of copper. From the x-ray diffraction patterns and electron probe microanalyses of the samples, it was found that, as the holding time increased, in 2.0% nitric acid or hydrochloric acid solutions, the HA phase of the pulverized granules had decomposed, and both calcium and phosphorus concentrations gradually decreased. After 3 hours of stirring, the pulverized granules

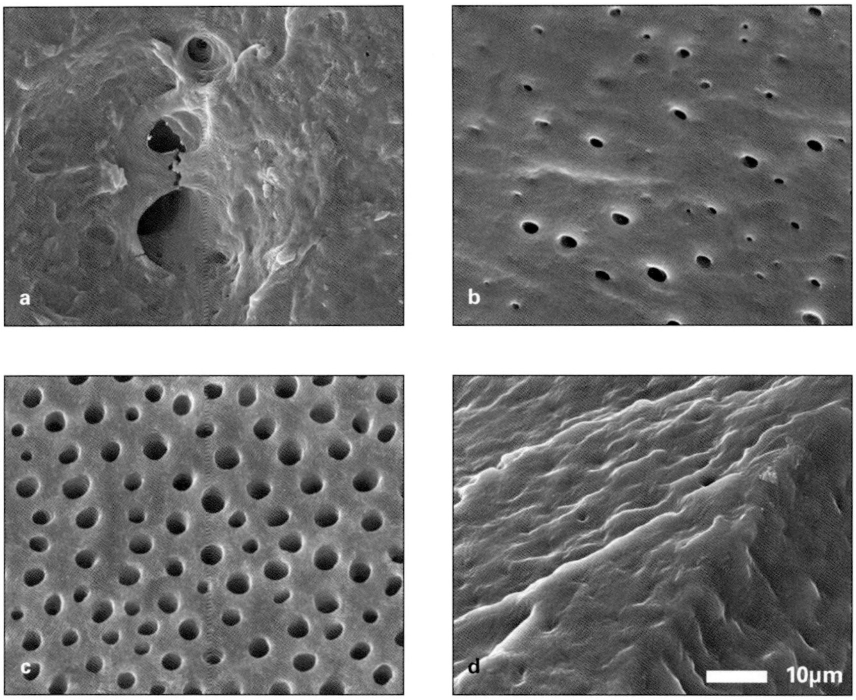

Fig 9-3 SEM images of DDM granules obtained by dissolution at 293 K and pH 1 for 3 hours under 500 rpm in various nitric acid solutions. *(a)* Microstructure of the DDM granules after dissolution in 0.3% nitric acid. *(b)* Microstructure of the DDM granules after dissolution in 0.5% nitric acid. *(c)* Microstructure of the DDM granules after dissolution in 1.0% nitric acid. *(d)* Microstructure of the DDM granules after dissolution in 2.0% nitric acid.

were completely demineralized and the weight had decreased to about one-fifth of its original.

Figure 9-3 shows SEM images of the DDM granules after being dissolved at room temperature under 500 rpm for 3 hours in 0.3% to 2.0% nitric acid aqueous solutions. In all cases, many dentinal tubules were observed in the DDM granules. With increasing concentrations of nitric acid, the crystallinity of HA decreased and the surfaces of the granules became rough because of elution of mineral components.[7] Moreover, following treatment with 0.3% to 2.0% hydrochloric acid solutions, a similar microstructure was observed, although the dissolution efficacy of the pulverized granules by nitric acid solutions was a little higher than that achieved by the hydrochloric acid solutions.[5]

Surface Modification of DDM Granules by a Specific Precipitation

To design new biomaterials with excellent selective adsorption for biopolymers and activation for osteoblasts or dental pulp, HA microcrystals were precipitated on partial or complete DDM granules. An HA nanocrystal coating, ie, surface modification of DDM granules, may help control the bioabsorption rate and osteoinductive ability of biomaterials, making them adaptable to any medical indication, depending on the coating conditions of the HA microcrystals.

The pH of the nitric acid demineralization solutions was carefully adjusted to less than 8.4 by dropwise addition of an ammonia aqueous solution to prevent denaturation of the collagen proteins. The sample slurries were aged by stirring at 298 K for 24 hours to synthesize HA-coated DDM granules. The functional DDM granules were filtered, washed with distilled water, freeze-dried or dried at room temperature for 24 hours, and stored at 277 K.[8]

Figure 9-4 shows SEM images of functional DDM granules prepared at 298 K in a pH of 7.0 to 8.4 for 24 hours after demineralization for 3 hours in 0.5% to 2.0% nitric acid aqueous solutions. HA nanocrystals (10 to 100 nm) were precipitated on the surfaces of DDM granules. The HA-coated films were more homogenous and dense for DDM granules with high demineralization efficiency, effected by dissolution in 2.0% nitric acid solution.[6]

The Brunauer-Emmett-Teller (BET)–specific surface areas were measured with nitrogen adsorption at 77 K. Curves of pore size distribution were calculated from the adsorption isotherms of nitrogen using the Cranston-Inkley equation and assuming a columnar pore model. The HA-coated DDM granules had much higher specific surface areas and total pore volumes.

Moreover, to improve surface activity of the DDM granules without denaturation of proteins, the surface structure of the DDM was modified in a biomimetic environment. Partial or complete DDM granules were soaked at 309.5 K and pH 7.4 in simulated body fluid (an inorganic aqueous solution with ion concentrations and pH nearly equal to those in human plasma).

Since the DDM had HA-forming ability in the solution that was supersaturated with respect to apatite, nanocrystals of

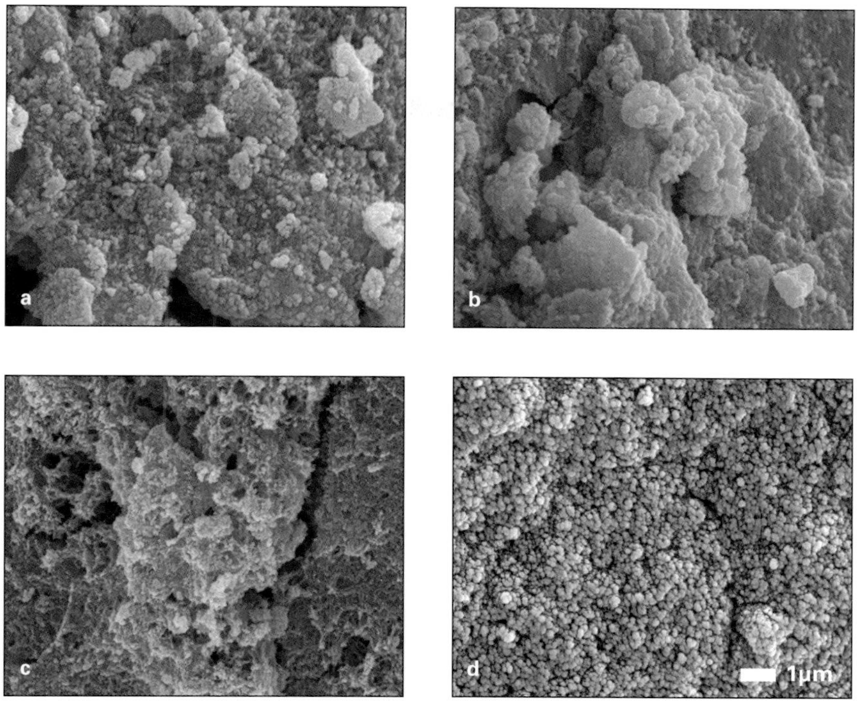

Fig 9-4 SEM photographs of functional DDM granules prepared at 298 K and pH 7.0 to 8.4 for 24 hours after demineralization for 3 hours in various nitric acid aqueous solutions. *(a)* Microstructure of HA-coated DDM granules obtained by freeze-drying (FD) after dissolution for 3 hours in 0.5% nitric acid. *(b)* Microstructure of HA-coated DDM granules obtained by FD after dissolution in 1.0% nitric acid. *(c)* Microstructure of HA-coated DDM granules obtained by FD after dissolution in 2.0% nitric acid. *(d)* Microstructure of HA-coated DDM granules obtained by static drying after dissolution in 2.0% nitric acid.

calcium phosphate were precipitated on surfaces of the DDM with increases in the soaking time. Different crystalline morphologies were observed, depending on the demineralization efficiency of the DDM. After 1 day of soaking, porous bone-like apatites were seen for the DDM with low demineralization efficiencies; after 6 days, fiber-oriented aggregates were recognized.[8]

Bioabsorption and Osteoinduction Characteristics of DDM Granules

The DDM and HA-coated granules, sterilized by ultraviolet irradiation, were implanted into the subcutaneous tissues of the back region in 4-week-old male nude mice. At 2 and 4 weeks after implantation, these samples were removed. In all procedures, the international guidelines for experiments on animals were followed.[2] The specimens were fixed in 10% neutral buffered formalin, decalcified with 10% formic acid, embedded in paraffin, sectioned, stained with hematoxylin-eosin, and observed under an optical microscope.

Infection and exclusion of the DDM granules were not observed. At 2 weeks after implantation, the granules showed a dense surface structure, and many dentinal tubules were covered by a thin fibrous film. At 4 weeks, Howship lacunae and osteoinduction were partially observed on the surface layers of the granules.[9] Hence, for HA-coated DDM granules, at 4 weeks, osteoinduction and bioabsorption by multiple giant cells, rather than inflammatory cell infiltration, were recognized on the surface layers of the granules.[7]

From these results, it is suggested that the DDM granules served as functional biomaterials controlling bioabsorption and osteoinduction and initiated bone formation because of their effective chemical composition.

Conclusion

A new cooling-pulverizing and processing technique that employed a small pulverizing apparatus produced new biomaterials, within a short time, that were adaptable to different therapeutic indications. With the apparatus, the authors designed pulverized granules of extracted human teeth to form DDM granules with excellent adsorption and release characteristics for growth factors by selecting the appropriate acid dissolution conditions. To provide functional control of the solid-liquid interface, HA microcrystals were easily coated on the surfaces of the DDM granules to increase the ability to adsorb biopolymer or cells.

These functional DDM granules, mixed with dental pulp, might be applied as innovative biomaterials for bone-regenerative therapy with autologous tissue for dental or advanced medical therapies, such as bone defects caused by periodontal disease, transplantation of teeth, and bone augmentation for implantation.

References

1. Akazawa T, Murata M, Takahata M, et al. Characterization of microstructure and bio-absorption of the hydroxyapatite ceramics modified by a partial dissolution-precipitation technique using supersonic treatment. J Ceram Soc Jpn 2010;118:535–540.
2. Murata M, Akazawa T, Arisue M. Bone engineering: Biological materials and bone morphogenetic proteins. Phosphorus Res Bull 2004;17:51–58.
3. Murata M, Akazawa T, Hino J, Tazaki J, Itoh K, Arisue M. Bone induction using human dematerialized dentin matrix and recombinant human BMP-2. Arch Bioceram Res 2005;5:178–181.
4. Murata M, Kawai T, Kawakami T, et al. Human acid-insoluble dentin with BMP-2 accelerates bone induction in subcutaneous and intramuscular tissues. J Ceram Soc Jpn 2010;118:438–441.
5. Akazawa T, Murata M, Nakamura K, et al. Preparation and characterization of demineralized dentin granules with osteoinduction originated from unnecessary human teeth. In: Shimabayashi (ed). Proceedings of the 16th Meeting on Inorganic Phosphorus Chemistry. Hiroshima: Letterpress, 2006:91–92.
6. Akazawa T, Murata M, Nakamura K, et al. Functional design of collagen/apatite composite granules derived from extraction of human teeth. In: Kanamura K (ed). Proceedings of Annual Meeting of the Ceramic Society of Japan. Hiroshima: Letterpress, 2007:132.
7. Akazawa T, Murata M, Hino J, et al. Materials design and application of demineralized dentin/apatite composite granules derived from human teeth. Arch Bioceram Res 2007;7:25–28.
8. Akazawa T, Murata M, Hino J, et al. Surface structure and biocompatibility of demineralized dentin matrix granules soaked in simulated body fluid. Appl Surface Sci 2012; 262:51–55.
9. Murata M, Akazawa T, Takahata M, et al. Bone induction of human tooth and bone crushed by newly developed automatic mill. J Ceram Soc Jpn 2010;118:434–437.

10

Autotransplantation of Teeth and Decalcified Dentin into the Atrophied Anterior Maxilla

Morihiro Kimura, Masaru Murata

Autotransplantation of teeth can now be performed in dental clinics. A host site for an autotransplanted tooth needs enough bone to stabilize the transplanted tooth in the drilled cavity. Buccal alveolar bone that is thin makes the extraction more difficult, and the buccal bone is therefore sometimes destroyed after the extraction. Moreover, following tooth loss, the jaw becomes atrophied physiologically. The present chapter reports on the application of an innovative therapy that combines ridge expansion and autografting with demineralized dentin matrix (DDM) for tooth autotransplantation.

Case Report

This patient was treated with extraction of all maxillary incisors and autotransplantation of the mandibular first premolars combined with DDM derived from third molars.

Presentation and diagnosis

A 42-year-old woman presented with deep caries of the maxillary right and left central incisors and left lateral incisor. Her medical history was unremarkable, and she did not smoke. The patient was concerned with the loss of retention of her maxillary incisors. The right central incisor showed a root fracture, and the deep caries rendered it hopeless as a possible abutment for partial dentures. The right and left central incisors and left lateral incisor were extracted, and wound healing proceeded very well. Clinical examination revealed a concave shape of the labial bone at 6 months after the extractions. Atrophy of the bone had taken place in the area of the maxillary incisors.

Surgical procedure

First, the nonfunctional maxillary left third molar was extracted to be transformed into DDM. The tooth was crushed with saline ice blocks in a newly developed mill (Osteomill, Tokyo Iken) for 30 seconds. The crushed tooth granules were decalcified completely in 0.03-N nitric acid solution for 20 minutes. The DDM granules were rinsed extensively in cold distilled water.[1] Wet DDM materials were obtained for immediate grafting.

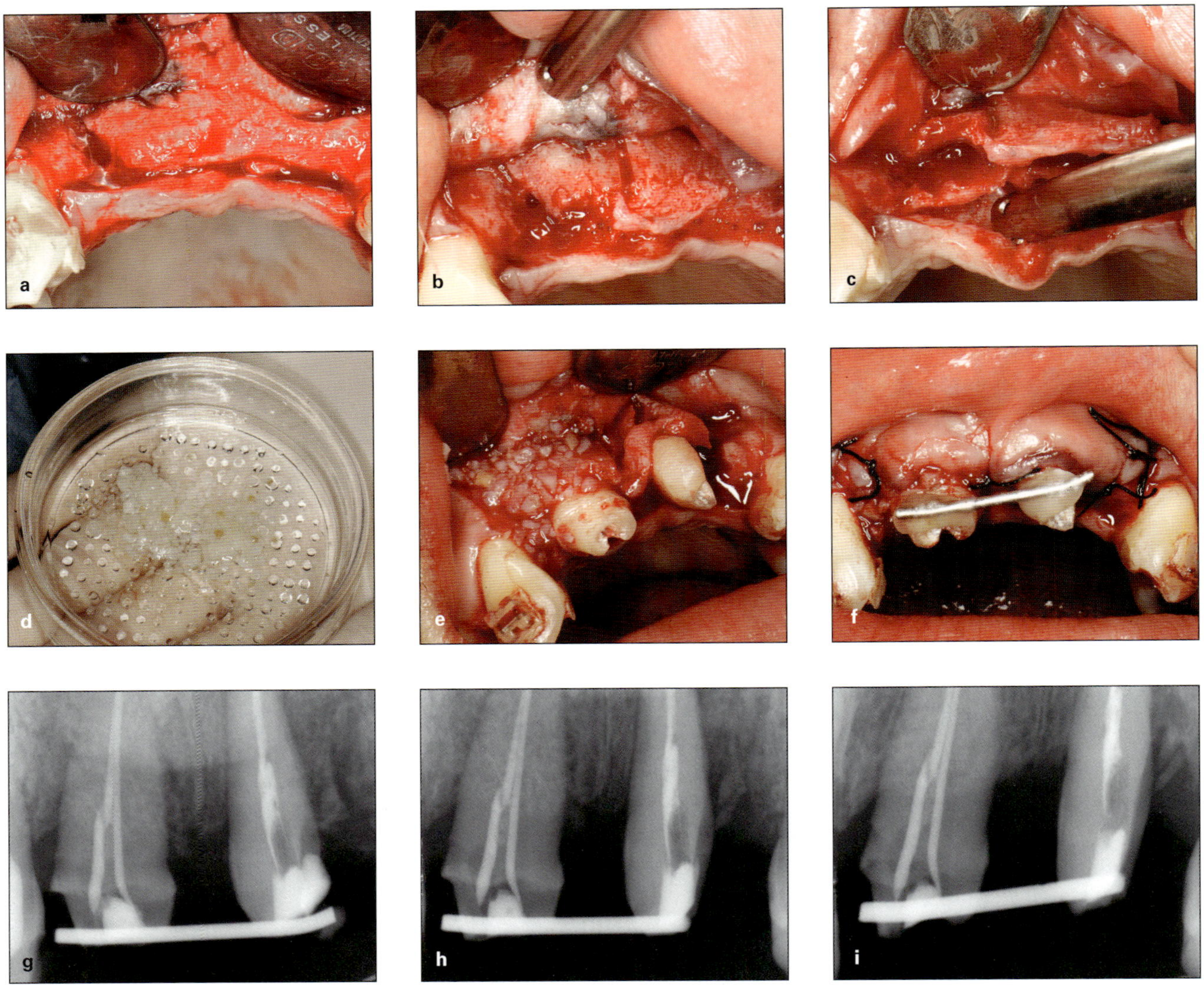

Fig 10-1 Surgical procedure with modified split osteotomy and autograft of teeth and DDM. *(a)* Frontal bone bed after flap elevation. Note the insufficient bone volume. *(b)* Formed grooves on the labial bone. *(c)* Transplanted spaces after ridge expansion. The right space is ready to receive the mandibular left first premolar, and the left space will receive the mandibular right first premolar. *(d)* DDM granules after demineralization in nitric acid for 20 minutes. *(e)* Autotransplantation of mandibular premolars and autograft of DDM granules prepared from the maxillary third molars. *(f)* Fixation with stainless bar and 4-methacryloxyethyl trimellitate anhydride. *(g)* Radiograph just after surgery. Note the immediate root canal filling. *(h)* Periapical radiograph 1 month after surgery. *(i)* View 12 months after surgery. Note the clear periodontal ligament space at the maxillary left central incisor.

After a flap had been elevated, a new minor osteotomy was performed for ridge expansion (Figs 10-1a). Briefly, two vertical grooves on the labial side and a groove on the top of the atrophied bone were formed with a bur under water cooling (Fig 10-1b). Next, the thin labial bone was expanded gently with a chisel in a greenstick fracture–like technique (Fig 10-1c). Osteotomies were created in the extended space between the labial and palatal plates large enough to fit tooth roots. The donor teeth (mandibular right and left first premolars) were extracted, and the root canals were filled immediately through the use of a tooth fixation device (Fix, Tokyo Iken). The roots, with their vital periodontal ligament cells, were placed gently into the cavities and covered with wet DDM (Figs 10-1d and 10-1e). The transplanted teeth were splinted together with a stainless bar and 4-methacryloxyethyl trimellitate anhydride adhesive on the coronal ends (Figs 10-1f and 10-1g).

Results and Discussion

Autotransplantation of two teeth and simultaneous placement of DDM successfully restored the patient's esthetic zone. The immediate grafting with DDM was carried out with a newly developed tooth mill.[1] Wet DDM was prepared about 30 minutes after the extractions and was transplanted immediately into the labial bone defect. Interestingly, compared with the radiographic view at 1 month after the procedure (Fig 10-1h), the periodontal ligament space was observed clearly at the periphery of the left transplanted tooth on a radiograph obtained at 12 months (Fig 10-1i). The authors believe that autogenous DDM contributed to the formation of biologic width around the labiolingual available bone. Human DDM induced bone and cartilage at 4 weeks after implantation in nude mice, and the acid-insoluble dentin (so-called DDM) was also recognized as a superior absorbable material for recombinant bone morphogenetic protein 2.[2]

Conclusion

The present adult patient was successfully restored with autotransplantation of teeth and DDM autograft. Immediate grafting with DDM was achieved using a newly developed mill. The DDM contributed to the regeneration of a labial bone defect and the biologic width as an innovative biomaterial.

References

1. Murata M, Akazawa T, Takahata M, et al. Bone induction of human tooth and bone crushed by newly developed automatic mill. J Ceram Soc Jpn 2010;118:434–437.
2. Murata M, Sato D, Hino J, et al. Acid-insoluble human dentin as carrier material for recombinant human BMP-2. J Biomed Mater Res A 2012;100:571–577.

11

Maxillary Bone Transport and Autologous Tooth Bone Grafting for Alveolar Cleft Repair

Masaharu Mitsug, Shingo Hara

Secondary autogenous cancellous bone grafting is a widely used method for the treatment of alveolar clefts and oronasal fistulae. Surgery for grafting the cleft maxilla and palate involves a procedure with three layers—an autogenous cancellous bone graft sandwiched between the nasal floor and the oral mucosa. An incision is made around the cleft to preserve the fixed gingiva to circumscribe the fistula. The tissue is then elevated from the bone on both sides of the cleft in the subperiosteal plane to the level of the anterior nasal spine and the lateral piriform rim. The tissue is elevated, inverted, and sutured to reconstruct the nasal floor. Fresh cancellous bone harvested from the iliac crest is condensed into the cleft defect and over the hypoplastic bone edges of the cleft. The soft tissue is either rotated or advanced to cover the bone grafts.[1]

Several autogenous donor sites have been used for alveolar bone grafting, including the iliac crest, rib, calvarium, tibia, and mandibular symphysis. Iliac crest bone is regarded as the gold standard for alveolar bone grafting but has disadvantages, such as the risk of prolonged postoperative pain, gait disturbances, a long hospital stay, unsightly scars, and/or sensory disturbances (neuropraxia of the lateral cutaneous nerve of the thigh).

Failure of iliac bone grafting sometimes occurs as a result of inadequate coverage of the graft with the surrounding soft tissue, pronounced scar formation, or large clefts. Maxillary bone transport can be a good solution when failure has occurred.[2] The method reported in this chapter has improved the oral environment in patients with cleft lip and palate, allowing orthodontic movement of teeth into the graft area and providing a stable foundation for orthodontic treatment. In this bone transport method, bone is distracted in the direction of the defect by osteotomy of bone adjacent to the defect, which allows for simultaneous distraction of the surrounding soft tissue. The total amount of bone grafted is small, and there is no donor site morbidity. Autologous tooth bone graft (ATBG) is a good grafting material. It avoids the need for a donor site; it promotes osteogenesis, osteoinduction, osteoconduction, and rapid healing; and it does not induce immune rejection.[3] The following case illustrates the application of the combination of maxillary bone transport and grafting with autogenous extracted teeth for alveolar cleft repair.[2]

Maxillary Bone Transport for Alveolar Cleft Repair

This method is indicated for patients with cleft lip, alveolus, and/or palate who have large untreated alveolar clefts, patients whose bone grafts have failed, those who have crowding and require space for dental correction, or patients who do not desire iliac bone grafting (Fig 11-1).

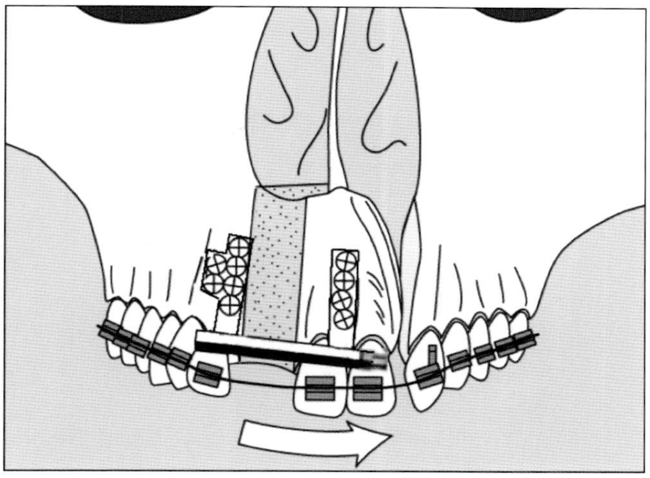

Fig 11-1 Illustration of original procedure for maxillary bone transport for alveolar cleft repair, which consists of alveolar bone transportation, closure of the alveolar cleft, and/or grafting of new bone. After a sagittal interdental osteotomy is extended to the nasal floor, the segmented alveolar bone is transported using a ready-made bone-supported distractor in combination with an orthodontic archwire. This method allows simultaneous correction of nasal septal deviation and maxillary arch deformities and malocclusion without donor sacrifice. After a consolidation period following distraction, a cancellous bone graft harvested from the new bone that has been created in the distraction gap is inserted at the docking site at the time of removal of the device. (Reprinted from Mitsugi et al[4] with permission.)

Before surgery, the local area is examined, and a study model and cephalograms are created and evaluated in detail. In addition, for three-dimensional (3D) evaluation of the dental arches, imaging diagnosis of the maxilla can be performed with 3D computed tomography (CT). The authors have used a vertical device for alveolar bone distraction (KLS Martin), which is fixed horizontally at the maxillary bone. Bone segment transport using the distractor is linear, but ideally, bone transportation along the curve of the dental arch is desirable. For this, an orthodontic archwire can be used as a "rail." A bracket is positioned to allow passive application of the wire. Using an indirect bonding method, the brackets are attached to a thin archwire. This allows movement of the dental arch together with the bracket along the curve of the wire.

The surgery can be performed under local anesthesia at an outpatient clinic. A minimal incision is made on the buccal side, and a buccal periosteal flap is raised, while the alveolar crest and palatal periosteum are preserved to maintain blood flow. A sagittal interdental osteotomy is performed completely to the nasal floor. The plate of the distractor is fixed with a screw, and the surgeon must take care to avoid contact with the dental root. After confirmation of the mobility of the bone segment, the wound is closed.

Distraction is performed after a period of 3 to 5 days. To avoid pressure on the gingiva, a rather slow distraction rate (0.3 to 0.5 mm/day) is used. At the end of the activation period, any extra soft tissue in the cleft can be removed using an electric knife to ensure close bone contact at the site where the anterior surface of the alveolar cleft comes into contact with the posterior surface of the alveolar cleft by maxillary bone transport.

After a consolidation period of 6 to 8 weeks after distraction, cancellous bone is grafted into the small space at the docking site under local anesthesia at the time of removal of the distraction device. Originally in this technique, grafting material was harvested from the new bone in the distraction gap.[2] The teeth are aligned by postoperative orthodontic treatment to guide them toward the distracted area. Tooth movement into the cleft area is initiated only after confirmation of the survival of the bone graft.

In patients with bilateral clefts, one side can be narrowed by dental arch correction, and bone grafting is performed. When this treatment is performed at an outpatient clinic, intraoral bone is used for grafting. Maxillary transport is initiated after 3 to 4 weeks, before adequate consolidation of the bone graft. The subsequent procedure is similar to that for patients with unilateral cleft.

Autologous Tooth Bone Grafting

After grafting, bone graft material should be replaced by bone that can withstand masticatory forces following remodeling and regrowth. Like alveolar bone, a tooth includes type I collagen, as well as hydroxyapatite, an essential component for bone remodeling. Therefore, autogenous teeth can be used as a novel bone graft material to replace damaged alveolar bone.[3] Commercially available bone substitutes have limitations, including a lack of osteoinductive and osteoconductive properties, a need for sterilization, and a risk of transmitting infectious disease. ATBG may be an ideal alternative to these grafting materials. ATBG contains organic and inorganic mineral components and is prepared from autogenous tissue, thus eliminating the risk of an immune reaction that may lead to rejection.

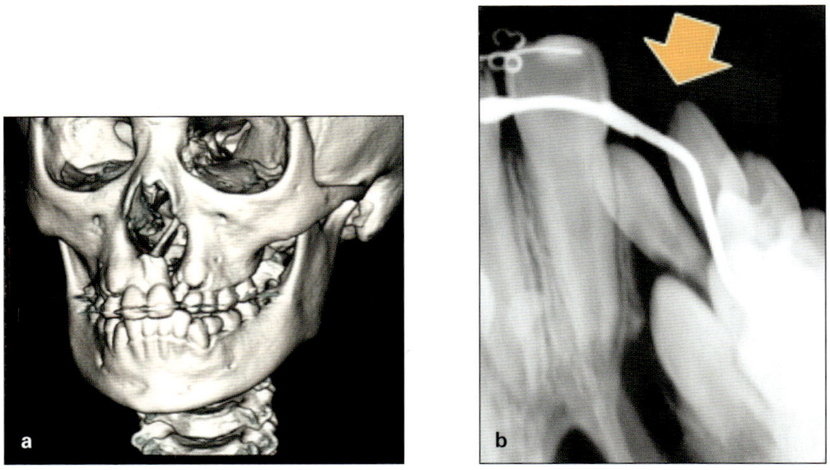

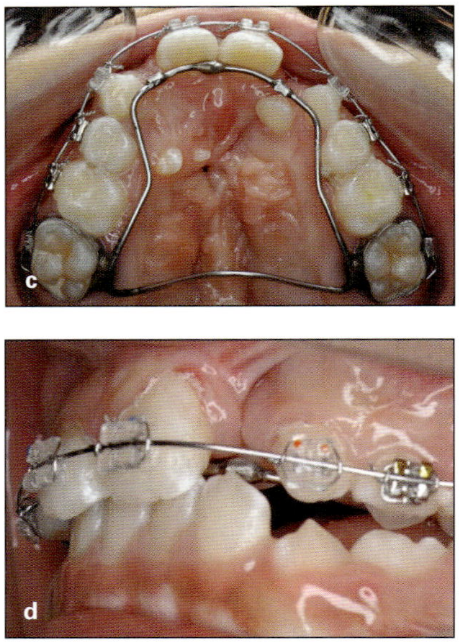

Fig 11-2 Treatment of a 9-year-old girl with distraction osteogenesis and ATBG. *(a)* Presurgical 3D CT showing the left-side alveolar cleft. *(b)* Presurgical occlusal radiograph showing the alveolar cleft on the left side. *(c,d)* Presurgical photographs showing the alveolar cleft and fistulae, the deviation of the maxillary midline, and the impaction of the left canine.

ATBG has already been used for bone grafting in implant surgery (such as maxillary sinus elevation or augmentation of the alveolar crest) and periodontal surgery and can be used in oral and maxillofacial surgery. By the end of 2011, more than 30,000 bone grafting procedures using ATBG had already been performed in Korea through the Korea Auto-Tooth and Bone Bank and at its related hospitals. Among these cases, 80% used a powder-type ATBG and 20% used a block type for implant surgery (eg, guided bone regeneration, sinus elevation). The frequency of wound rupture and infection in patients treated with ATBG was the same as that in other cases using other synthetic grafting materials; however, complete loss of an ATBG has never been reported.[5] The use of ATBG, which is produced from each patient's own teeth, results in excellent bone healing, most likely as a result of its inorganic components and surface structure. Histologic analysis of the healing process in harvested specimens after clinical application has provided further evidence of success with this material.

Patient Report

A 9-year-old girl suffering from unilateral (left-sided) cleft lip and palate was treated with this method. She had undergone labioplasty at 6 months of age and palatoplasty at age 1.5 years of age. However, a deviation of the upper midline from the facial midline was still present, and the alveolar cleft and fistulae (left side) remained. The maxillary left canine was impacted in an apicodistal position (Figs 11-2a to 11-2d). Maxillary bone transport using a virtual operation with SimPlant OMS (Materialise Dental) was planned to repair the alveolar cleft and to correct the maxillary midline and deviated nasal septum (Fig 11-2e).

Surgery was performed under local anesthesia with intravenous sedation. A sagittal interdental maxillary osteotomy was performed on the right side, between the maxillary incisors, and was extended completely to the nasal floor. Alveolar maxillary bone (above the central incisors) would be transported left using an alveolar distractor (TRACK 1.0, KLS Martin) to close the alveolar cleft (Fig 11-2f).

At the end of the transporter activation period, so-called docking-site surgery was performed to remove the soft tissue from the cleft using an electric knife; this ensured close bone contact at the docking site (Fig 11-2g). Two maxillary supernumerary teeth and a small left lateral incisor were extracted to be converted into ATBG (Figs 11-2h and 11-2i). The bone transporter was removed, and ATBG placement at the docking area was done simultaneously (Figs 11-2j to 11-2n).

Surgical closure of the alveolar cleft and fistulae was accomplished fairly simply through two surgeries under local anesthesia without complications, and good positioning of the maxillary canine was achieved with postoperative orthodontic treatment (Figs 11-2o to 11-2r). Maxillary bone transport allowed simultaneous correction of the nasal septal deviation and maxillary arch deformities and malocclusion, since the dental arch was expanded without the need for a donor site or soft tissue expansion. Placement of ATBG at the docking site allowed the repair of any remaining bone defect of the nasal floor and alveolar bone.

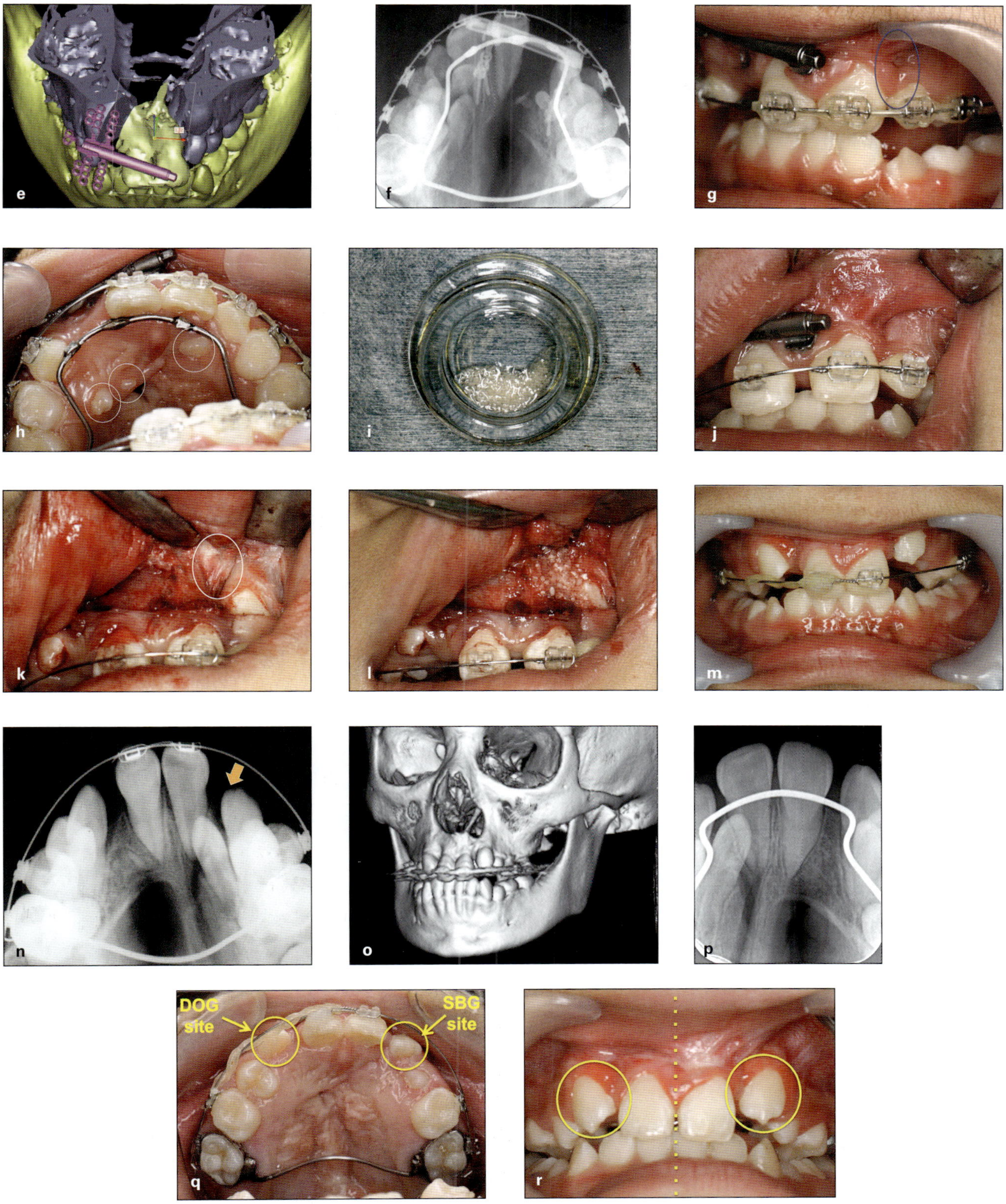

Fig 11-2 *(cont) (e)* Virtual surgery is done with SimPlant OMS using a Martin distractor to correct the maxillary midline and deviated nasal septum. *(f)* Radiograph during active distraction. *(g)* After the completion of maxillary bone distraction, 1 week after docking surgery. *(h)* The two supernumerary teeth and small left lateral incisor that will be used for ATBG are still in place *(circles)*. *(i)* The ATBG includes both enamel and dentin made into 0.16 g of powder-form material. *(j)* After 3 months of consolidation, good soft tissue healing is observed, but the alveolar bone contour is poor. *(k)* The bone defect cleft area *(circle)* at the docking site. *(l)* Placement of ATBG in the docking area. *(m)* Postsurgical intraoral view. *(n)* Postsurgical radiograph showing excellent repair of the alveolar cleft on the left side *(arrow)*. *(o)* At 1 year postoperative, a 3D CT shows a good result from the alveolar cleft repair (left side) and distraction osteogenesis (right side). *(p)* Radiograph showing the alveolar cleft repair. *(q,r)* Correction of the maxillary midline was carried out with elastics under the care of the orthodontist. Postsurgical intraoral photographs show that the maxillary canines are erupting properly at the distraction osteogenesis (DOG) site and at the secondary bone grafting (SBG) site.

Discussion

Conventional iliac crest bone grafting for the repair of alveolar clefts is associated with morbidity and a number of complications, such as a long hospital stay with surgery under general anesthesia, prolonged postoperative pain, and unsightly scars. Iliac crest bone harvesting also often interferes with a patient's schooling and may limit participation in sporting activities. The reported complication rate following iliac crest bone graft harvesting is 19.37%,[6] and the complication rate following iliac bone grafting into alveolar clefts is between 12.5% and 20%.[7,8]

The advantages of bone grafting using ATBG are that there is no need for autogenous donor sites (including iliac crest, rib, calvarium, tibia, and mandibular symphysis), and graft failures caused by infection and wound rupture are greatly reduced. Extracted primary teeth can be useful for ATBG, if preserved. However, combination of ATBG with maxillary distraction osteogenesis can further delay the timing of bone grafting for alveolar cleft. Third molars or premolars that have been extracted prior to orthodontic treatment may be recycled, if preserved. The disadvantages of bone grafting using ATBG include a limited number of teeth for extraction. However, the use of distraction can reduce the volume of ATBG required.

The combination of maxillary bone transport and bone grafting using ATBG for alveolar cleft repair can be performed in a few operations simply under local anesthesia, without the need for hospitalization. This treatment for alveolar cleft repair represents a good alternative to traditional approaches.

References

1. Turvey TA, Ruiz RL, Vig KWL, Costello BJ. Orthognathic surgery in the patient with cleft palate. In: Miloro M, Ghalia GE, Larsen PE, Waite PD (eds). Peterson's Principles of Oral and Maxillofacial Surgery, ed 2. Hamilton, ON: BC Decker 2004:1267–1275.
2. Mitsugi M, Ito M, Alcalde RE. Maxillary bone transportation in alveolar cleft-transport distraction osteogenesis for treatment of alveolar cleft repair. Br J Plast Surg 2005;58:619–625.
3. Kim YK, Kim SG, Byeon JH, et al. Development of a novel bone grafting material using autogenous teeth. Oral Surg Oral Med Oral Pathol Oral Radiol Endod 2010;109:496–503.
4. Mitsugi M, Um IW, Kim YK, Mim KW, Minamizato T, Murata M. Autotooth bone graft [in Japanese]. Quintessence 2013;32(12): 181–198.
5. Mitsugi M, et al. Novel bone grafting system using extracted autogenous teeth [in Japanese]. Quintessence 2011;30(6):87–95.
6. Dimitriou R, Mataliotakis GI, Angoules AG, Kanakaris NK, Giannoudis PV. Complications following autologous bone graft harvesting from the iliac crest and using the RIA: A systematic review. Injury 2011;42(suppl 2):S3–S15.
7. Perry CW, Lowenstein A, Rothkopf DM. Ambulatory alveolar bone grafting. Plast Reconstr Surg 2005;116:736–739.
8. Sindet-Pedersen S, Enemark H. Reconstruction of alveolar clefts with mandibular or iliac crest bone grafts: A comparative study. J Oral Maxillofac Surg 1990;48:554–558.

12

Maxillary Implant Restoration with Autograft of Decalcified Dentin Matrix

Yoji Kamiura, Ryuichiro Kumazawa, Takaki Kumazawa, Masaru Murata, Toshiyuki Akazawa

Extracted teeth are usually discarded as potentially infectious medical waste. However, the dental community is now considering human primary and secondary teeth as a useful resource for patients and their families. Highly calcified tissues such as cortical bone and dentin do not perform better in both osteoinduction and bone formation than spongy bone, decalcified bone matrix (DBM), and decalcified dentin matrix (DDM).[1] Dentin and bone are mineralized tissues and similar in their chemical components. Both DDM and DBM are composed of predominantly type I collagen (95%); the remaining material is made up of noncollagenous proteins, including a small amount of growth factors.[2] In other words, DDM and DBM can include acid-insoluble collagen-binding bone morphogenetic proteins (BMPs) along with several growth factors.[3,4] Human DDM has been shown to be capable of osteoinduction and to serve as a suitable carrier for BMP-2.[5]

Case Report

Presentation and diagnosis

A 28-year-old woman presented with a nonvital fractured tooth (the maxillary right central incisor). Her medical history was unremarkable, and she was a nonsmoker. The gingival margin of the fractured tooth was about 1 mm apical to that of the left central incisor (Figs 12-1a and 12-1b). Clinical examination revealed a V-shaped bone defect on the labial side of the nonvital right incisor. The final diagnosis was root fracture of the maxillary right central incisor accompanied by a labial alveolar bone defect.

First surgery

The fractured root was extracted gently using a periotome. The socket was filled with a collagenous sponge (Terplug, Olympus Terumo Biomaterials) and covered with an autogenous graft of mucoconnective tissue harvested from the palate for socket preservation under local anesthesia (Fig 12-1c). Computed tomography (CT) scans taken after surgery confirmed the labial bone loss (Figs 12-1d and 12-1e). A provisional crown was placed, since the affected area was in the esthetic zone.

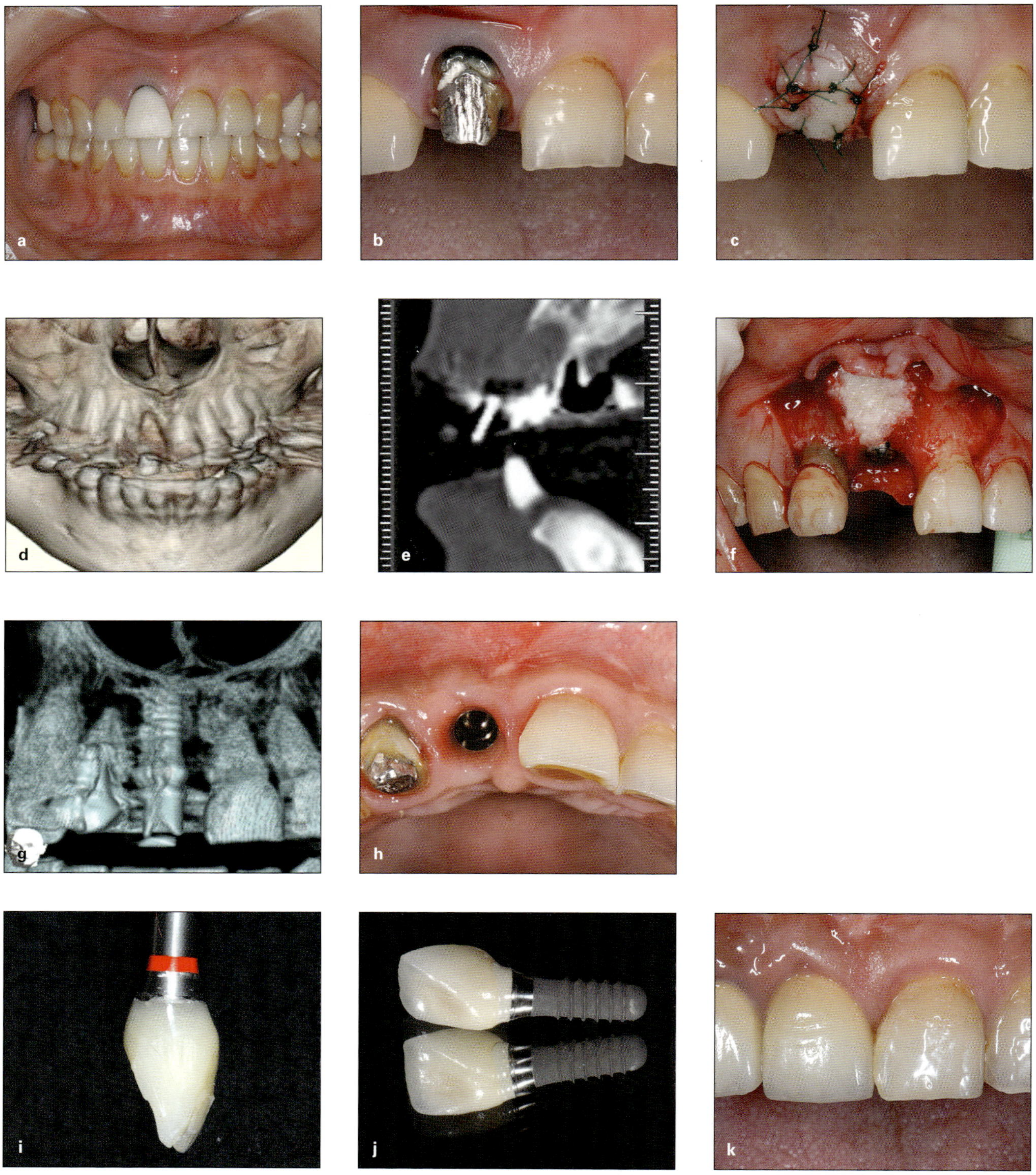

Fig 12-1 A 28-year-old woman with root fracture and labial alveolar bone defect on the maxillary right central incisor. *(a)* Initial appearance. *(b)* Gingival recession in the area of the fractured incisor. Note the inharmonious gingival margin. *(c)* A mucoconnective tissue autograft was placed for socket preservation. *(d)* Three-dimensional CT image showing the V-shaped labial bone defect. *(e)* Sagittal CT image showing labial bone loss. *(f)* Immediate autograft of DDM granules for bone regeneration. *(g)* CT image showing appropriate placement of the implant and grafting material. *(h)* Gingival profile around the implant. *(i)* Provisional restoration. Note the clearance that has been adjusted to avoid excessive pressure on the labial side. *(j)* Definitive zirconium crowns (Kavo Everest). *(k)* Final view after cementing the definitive restorations. Note the harmonized gingival margin and crown color.

Second surgery

At 8 weeks after the first surgery, a commercially pure titanium implant was placed, along with simultaneous autografting with DDM, under local anesthesia. First, the nonfunctional maxillary left third molar was extracted to be processed into DDM. The tooth was crushed with saline ice blocks in a tooth mill (Osteomill, Tokyo Iken) at 12,000 rpm for 30 seconds. The crushed tooth granules were decalcified completely in 0.026-N nitric acid solution for 20 minutes. The DDM granules were then extensively rinsed in cold distilled water[6,7] and were available for immediate transplantation about 30 minutes after extraction. Next, a titanium implant (Straumann Regular Neck implant with a diameter of 4.1 mm and length of 10 mm) was placed into the preserved socket, and DDM granules were grafted into the remaining bone defect around the implant (Fig 12-1f). CT scans were taken immediately after the surgery (Figs 12-1g and 12-1h).

A provisional crown was used for 3 months after implant placement (Fig 12-1i). The definitive prosthetic restorations were placed onto the implant and the right lateral incisor at 9 months after implantation and DDM transplantation (Fig 12-1j). The patient was very satisfied with the harmonized gingival margin and the ceramic crown color (Fig 12-1k).

Results and discussion

DDM granules were received without complications, and the biologic width was successfully established. This patient was successfully restored with a dental implant and a DDM autograft. The authors believe that the autogenous DDM material had contributed partially to establishing the biologic width of the labiolingual available bone. Immediate grafting with DDM can be achieved with the newly developed tooth mill.

Conclusion

The young adult patient was successfully restored with a single implant and DDM autograft. DDM granules from a vital tooth are highly insoluble collagenous matrices with osteoinductive potential. The DDM contributed to regeneration of the labial bone defect and the biologic width as an innovative biomaterial.

References

1. Huggins C, Wiseman S, Reddi AH. Transformation of fibroblasts by allogeneic and xenogeneic transplants of demineralized tooth and bone. J Exp Med 1970;132:1250–1258.
2. Finkelman RD, Mohan S, Jennings JC, Taylor AK, Jepsen S, Baylink DJ. Quantitation of growth factors IGF-I, SGF/IGF-II, and TGF-β in human dentin. J Bone Miner Res 1990;5:717–723.
3. Akazawa T, Murata M, Hino J, et al. Materials design and application of demineralized dentin/apatite composite granules derived from human teeth. Arch Bioceram Res 2007;7:25–28.
4. Murata M, Akazawa T, Tazaki J, et al. Human dentin autograft for bone regeneration—Automatic pulverizing machine and biopsy. Bioceramics 2009;22:745–748.
5. Murata M, Sato D, Hino J, et al. Acid-insoluble human dentin as carrier material for recombinant human BMP-2. J Biomed Mater Res A 2012;100:571–577.
6. Murata M, Kawai T, Kawakami T, et al. Human acid-insoluble dentin with BMP-2 accelerates bone induction in subcutaneous and intramuscular tissues. J Ceram Soc Jpn 2010;118:438–441.
7. Murata M, Akazawa T, Takahata M, et al. Bone induction of human tooth and bone crushed by newly developed automatic mill. J Ceram Soc Jpn 2010;118:434–437.

13

Extraction Socket Preservation and Reconstruction

Myung-Jin Kim, Young-Kyun Kim

A clean extraction socket will undergo normal healing. If an implant will be placed in 2 to 3 months, no special treatment of the socket is necessary. However, if implant treatment will be delayed or general prosthetic treatment is planned, resorption of alveolar bone is inevitable as time passes. Severe resorption of alveolar bone will cause problems, especially in the anterior arches, where esthetics are crucial. If progressive periodontal disease or an inflammatory lesion in the tooth root leads to severe defects on the surrounding bone wall after extraction, normal healing will not occur, since the soft tissues are depressed into the defect. In such cases, it is advisable to perform extraction socket preservation or reconstruction.

Resorption of the remaining alveolar bone around the extraction socket generally occurs soon after extraction and is more pronounced for teeth with periodontal disease. Tan et al[1] reported rapid bone loss in the first 3 to 6 months after tooth extraction followed by gradual resporption. Resorption after extraction makes it difficult to place implants and interferes with prosthetic treatment and oral hygiene. Many scholars recommend alveolar ridge preservation through placement of bone grafting material in extraction sockets, even if implant treatment is not planned.

There have been various attempts to preserve the alveolar ridge and minimize bone resorption. Alternative bonelike grafting materials, such as hard tissue replacement (HTR) polymer, bovine bone substitute (eg, Bio-Oss, Geistlich Biomaterials), demineralized freeze-dried bone, bioactive glass, and bovine hydroxyapatite (HA), and other materials, such as collagen and polylactic/polyglycolic acid sponge, have been used alone or together. Darby et al[2] concluded that alveolar ridge preservation should be performed after extraction if the thickness of the buccal cortical plate is less than 1.5 to 2.0 mm, if there are major anatomical structures near the extraction site (eg, maxillary sinus or inferior alveolar canal), if the site is in the esthetic zone, or if several teeth are extracted.

However, there have been conflicting findings about extraction socket preservation after extraction. Rothamel et al[3] studied extraction socket preservation using nanocrystal bovine HA paste and reported that alveolar ridge preservation was not effective because of unexpected resorption. Becker et al[4] suggested that the application of bone graft materials in a fresh extraction socket may be problematic, as the materials can interfere with the healing process of the extraction socket itself or that of an implant.

Various mixtures of bone graft materials and other materials have been introduced to maximize the effect of alveolar ridge preservation and improve bone formation. Shi et al[5] reported that the application of platelet-rich plasma with bone graft in extraction sockets improved alveolar ridge preservation and bone formation. Lekovic et al[6] reported that covering the extraction socket with a resorptive membrane after extraction could preserve the alveolar ridge. Neiva et al[7] reported that, when putty-type HA material and synthetic peptide P-15 were applied to alveolar ridges after maxillary premolar extraction, almost no change took place in the height of the alveolar ridge, with an average loss of 0.15 ± 1.76 mm after 4 months, whereas the control group, which did not receive the P-15, saw a mean decrease in ridge height of 0.56 ± 1.04 mm. However, in both groups, the alveolar ridge lost width—1.43 ± 1.05 mm for the control group and 1.31 ± 0.96 mm for the experimental group—with no statistically significant difference between the groups. Luczyszyn et al[8] reported that using bovine HA and acellular dermal matrix together could increase the diameter of keratinized tissues and improve the effect of alveolar ridge preservation. Iasella et al[9] performed ridge preservation using freeze-dried bone allograft and collagen membranes. Greater height and diameter of the alveolar ridge were achieved compared with untreated extraction sites. Sclar[10] introduced the Bio-Col method, in which the extraction socket is filled with Bio-Oss, covered with resorptive collagen sponge (Collaplug, Zimmer Dental), and equipped with a denture or a false tooth to induce spontaneous epithelialization of the extraction socket. Gross[11] used HTR polymer to fill the socket up to 1 mm apical to the alveolar crest, covered the top with Gelfoam (Pfizer), and completed primary closure using a local flap. Camargo et al[12] presented the results of a study of alveolar ridge preservation in which bioactive glass was placed after extraction, the socket was covered with calcium sulfate, and the open socket approach was applied. The authors found that internal fill-in was more prominent and less resorption was seen with regard to the height of the alveolar bone, but the width of the alveolar ridge was not very well preserved.

Darby et al[2] felt that it was valuable to fill extraction sockets with slow-absorbing osteoconductive bone graft materials and cover the top with resorptive membranes, as alveolar ridge preservation using Collaplug alone was not very effective. They stated that this method preserved the shape and amount of alveolar bone, and results would be favorable if implants were placed within 4 to 6 months. Serino et al[13] filled extraction sockets with polylactic/polyglycolic acid sponge and reported good clinical and histologic results. Kim et al[14] reported good alveolar ridge preservation and early bone formation in a clinical study of alveolar ridge preservation with gelatin sponge and platelet-rich plasma after extraction.

Artzi et al[15] filled human extraction sockets with anorganic bovine bone and analyzed the results clinically and histomorphometrically after 9 months. Inorganic components from the bovine bone material did not resorb until 9 months later, and lamellar bone increased and connective tissues decreased as new bone formation increased from the alveolar bone to the apex of the socket. Researchers have sought to determine whether implants can undergo osseointegration directly, before the remaining bone graft materials resorb, when inorganic materials such as bovine bone are used for extraction socket preservation and implantation. There have been conflicting findings. Valentini[16] and Hämmerle et al[17] reported no problems with osseointegration, whereas Becker et al[4] felt that these inorganic materials may interfere with osseointegration.

Clinical Study

The autogenous tooth bone graft material (ATBGM) developed by the authors has been known to have good biocompatibility, to heal by osteoinduction and osteoconduction, and to be resorbed after a certain period of time. In many cases, good extraction socket preservation and bone healing were seen when ATBGM was used alone or with resorbable membranes, verifying that this technique is suitable for extraction socket preservation. There may be differences in various clinical situations, but implants were successfully placed 2 months after extraction socket preservation was performed with ATBGM, and bone healing and reconstruction occurred quickly.

The authors surveyed the clinical results of extraction socket preservation procedures performed with ATBGM after extraction at Bundang Seoul National University Hospital's dental and periodontal departments between October 2008 and August 2009. The patients were, on average, 45.8 ± 8.4 years old; 8 were men and 10 were women. The teeth treated were 1 maxillary molar and 17 mandibular molars, all of which had two- or three-wall defects. The teeth were extracted using local anesthesia, and complete curettage was performed prior to filling the wounds with powder-form ATBGM. Resorbable membranes were used for coverage in nine sites (BioGide [Geistlich] in eight, Ossix Plus [Datum Dental] in one) and sutured into place, and the remaining nine sockets were left uncovered. In four patients, implants were successfully placed after 4 to 6 months of healing. Clinical and radiologic evaluations after extraction socket preservation revealed no complications (ie, infection), and the ATBGM tended to be resorbed and become new bone, with a bone density similar to that of the neighboring teeth.

Case Reports

Patient 1

A 60-year-old man with controlled diabetes presented with mobility and pain in the mandibular right second molar. He had a poor periodontal condition, and the roots of the maxillary left second molar and mandibular left first molar remained in situ (Fig 13-1a). The authors planned to extract the mandibular right second molar, perform periodontal treatment in both arches, and place a bone graft to support an implant after a certain healing period.

The maxillary left second molar roots were extracted, and scaling and root planing were performed in both arches. The mandibular left first and third molar roots were extracted, prepared, and stored as powder-type ATBGM. The mandibular right second molar was then extracted, prepared, and stored as powder-type ATBGM (Fig 13-1b). A month later, a mucoperiosteal flap was elevated in the mandibular right second molar area. The powder-type ATBGM was placed, the area was covered with a resorbable collagen membrane (BioGide),

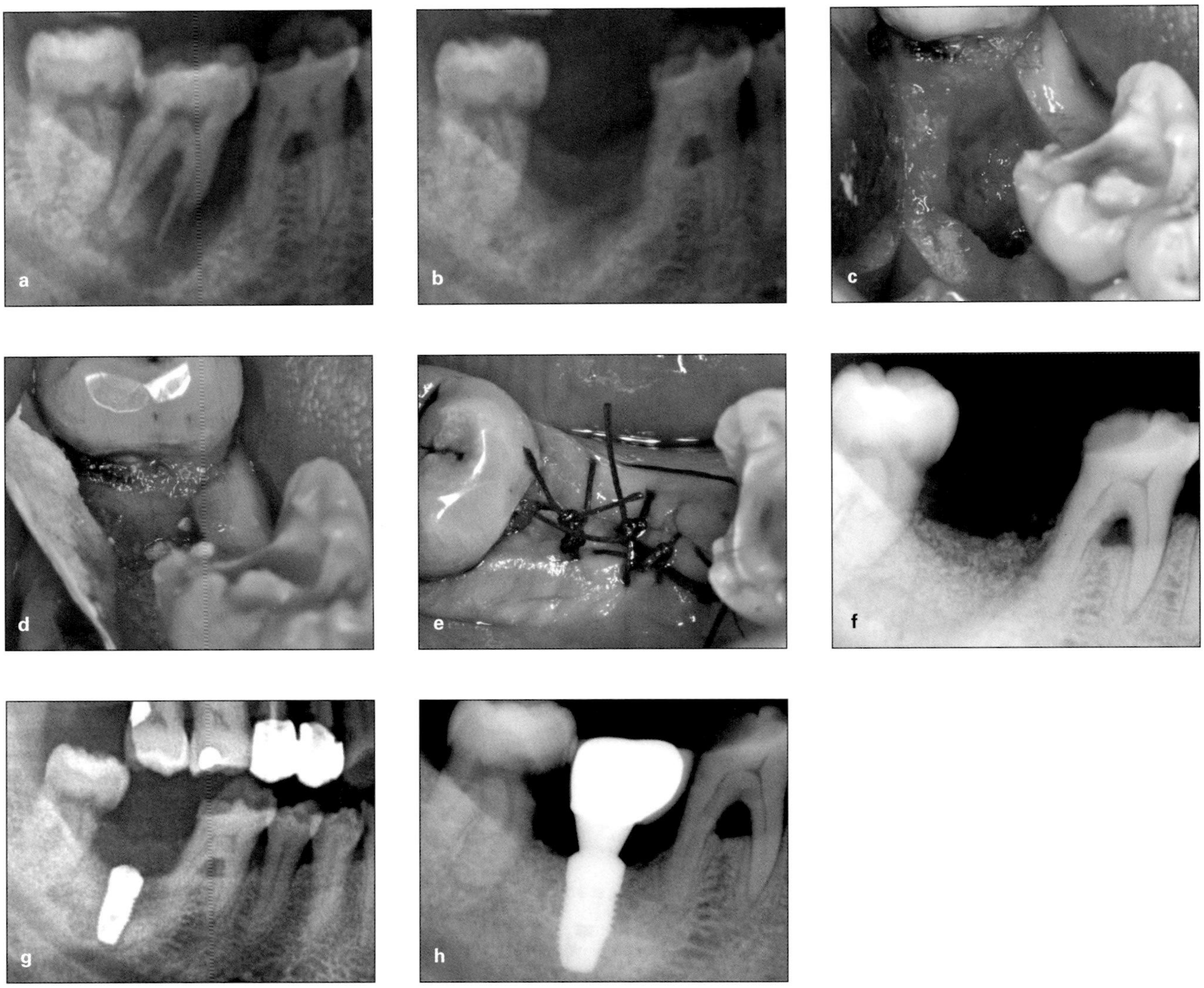

Fig 13-1 *(a)* At initial diagnosis, the periapical and periodontal inflammatory lesions on the mandibular right second molar were very close to the inferior alveolar canal. *(b)* After the extraction of the mandibular right second molar. *(c)* Elevation of a mucoperiosteal flap. *(d)* ATBGM in place and covered with a resorbable membrane. *(e)* The wound has been sutured. *(f)* Periapical radiograph 3 weeks after bone graft placement in the extraction socket. *(g)* After implant placement. *(h)* Periapical radiograph 4 months after restoration. (Courtesy of Prof Hyo Jeong Lee, Seoul, Korea.)

and the wound was sutured (Figs 13-1c to 13-1f). The site was allowed to heal for 6 months before a 4.8 × 10–mm implant (Implantium) was placed in this area (Fig 13-1g). The bone quality was considered equivalent to D1, as assessed during drilling. Stage-two surgery was performed 4 months later, and a maxillary prosthesis was placed after 3 more months of healing (Fig 13-1h).

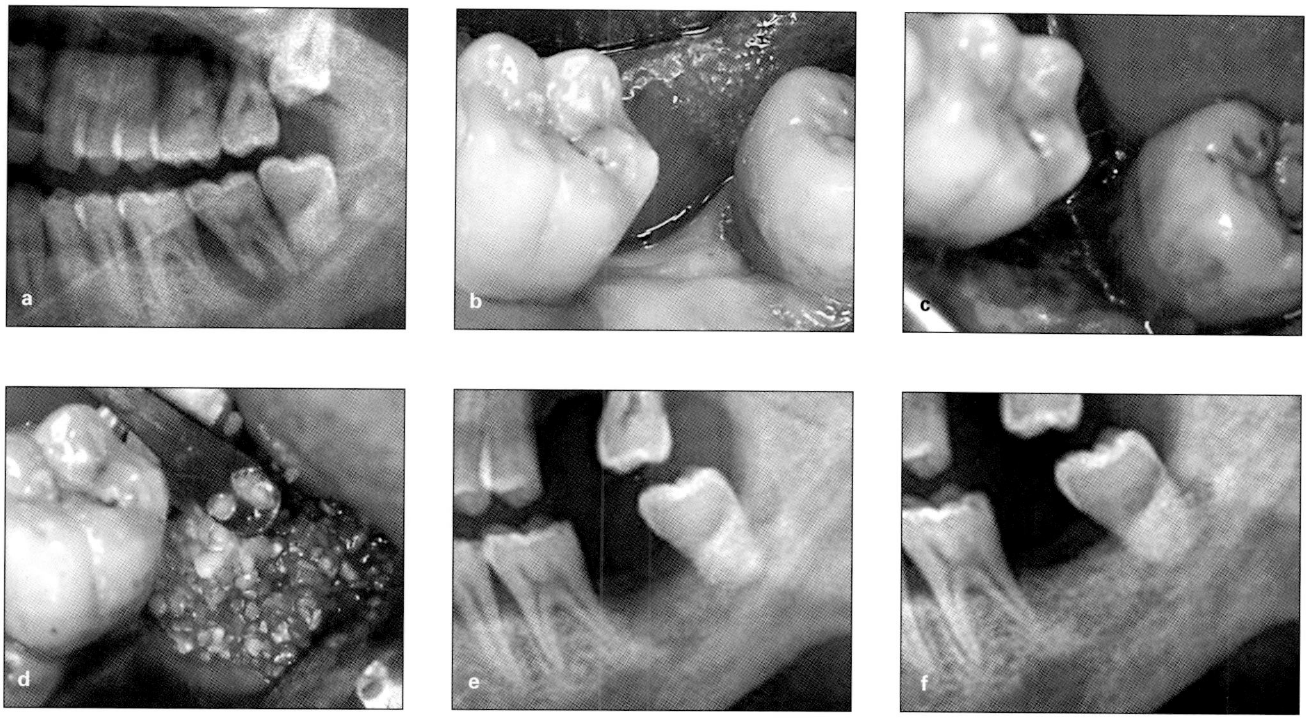

Fig 13-2 *(a)* At initial diagnosis, the periapical inflammatory lesion on the mandibular left second molar was very close to the inferior alveolar canal. *(b)* At 2 months after extraction of the mandibular left second molar. *(c)* Elevation of a mucoperiosteal flap revealed that the extraction socket had healed incompletely. *(d)* Powder-type ATBGM in place. *(e)* Immediately after bone grafting. *(f)* At 5 months after bone grafting, the alveolar bone height was stable and bone healing was almost perfect. (Courtesy of Prof Hyo Jeong Lee, Seoul, Korea.)

Patient 2

A 36-year-old man presented with gingival swelling and pain in the mandibular left second molar area and generalized tooth mobility (Fig 13-2a). Chronic periodontitis was diagnosed, and extraction and implant placement were planned.

The mandibular left second molar was extracted, and complete periapical curettage was performed to induce natural healing of the extraction socket. The extracted tooth was processed into powder-type ATBGM for storage. After 2 months of healing, a mucoperiosteal flap was elevated for implant placement; however, the extraction socket had not healed completely, and the inferior alveolar nerve could have been damaged if an implant was placed before healing was complete (Figs 13-2b and 13-2c). Granulation tissues were removed from the extraction socket, ATBGM was placed in the socket (Figs 13-2d and 13-2e), the area was covered with resorbable collagen membrane (BioGide), and the wound was sutured. Periodontal treatment was performed in both arches during the healing period, and the maxillary left first and third molars were extracted. Five months later, it was apparent that the height of the alveolar bone in the mandibular left second molar region was very stable (Fig 13-2f).

Patient 3

A 53-year-old woman presented with a mobile mandibular left first molar (Fig 13-3a). Clinical and radiologic examinations revealed that she had clinical periodontitis, with several teeth lost and serious bone loss around the molar in question. Extraction of the mobile tooth for processing into ATBGM was planned to enable reconstruction of the defects in the extraction socket and implant placement.

The mandibular left first molar was extracted, and periapical curettage was performed. The extracted tooth was processed into ATBGM and stored. After 6 weeks of healing, a mucoperiosteal flap was elevated in the area (Fig 13-3b); ATBGM was placed, the area was covered with a resorbable collagen membrane (BioGide) (Fig 13-3c), and the wound was sutured. Very successful bone healing was apparent upon clinical and radiologic examinations 4 months later (Fig 13-3d).

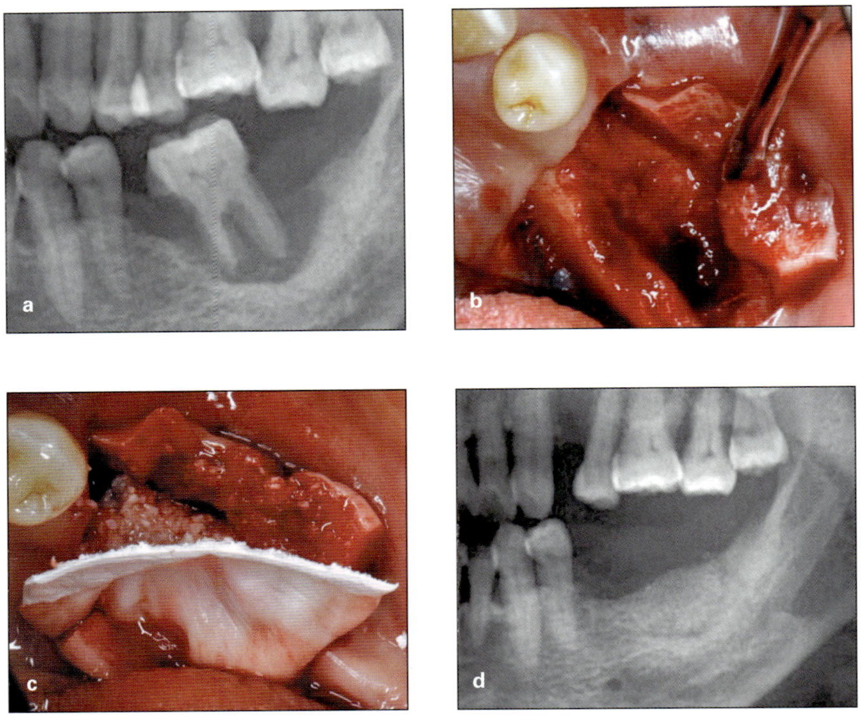

Fig 13-3 *(a)* At initial diagnosis. Very serious bone loss had occurred around the mandibular left first molar, and natural healing after extraction could not be expected without special treatment. *(b)* Elevation of a mucoperiosteal flap revealed that the extraction socket had barely healed. *(c)* Powder-form ATBGM in place and covered with a resorbable membrane. *(d)* At 4 months after bone grafting, the height of alveolar bone was perfectly maintained and bone healing was very successful. (Courtesy of Prof Hyo Jeong Lee, Seoul, Korea.)

Patient 4

A 45-year-old man presented with a mobile mandibular right second molar (Fig 13-4a). Clinical and radiologic examinations revealed buccal gingival swelling and a radiolucent lesion with severe destruction of alveolar bone around the mobile tooth. Chronic periodontitis and periodontal abscess were diagnosed. It was decided to extract the tooth and perform extraction socket preservation using ATBGM, as there was insufficient bone between the socket and the inferior alveolar canal.

The mandibular right second molar was extracted and processed into ATBGM in powder (crown) and block (root) forms. Two weeks later, the granulation tissues were removed from the extraction socket, the block and powder were placed, the area was covered with resorbable collagen membrane (BioGide), and the wound was sutured (Figs 13-4b to 13-4h).

Five months after bone grafting (Fig 13-4i), an implant (Implantium Superline, 4.8D/6D/8L; implant stability quotient [ISQ] of 75) was placed in the area, and the wound was sutured (Figs 13-4j and 13-4k). The bone was rated as D2 in quality. Stage-two surgery was performed 5 months later, and the implant was at 85 ISQ (Fig 13-4l). The mandibular prosthesis was then restored (Fig 13-4m).

Patient 5

A patient presented with chronic periapical abscess around both mandibular second molars and an inflammatory lesion that had spread to the inferior alveolar canal (Fig 13-5a). Extraction of both mandibular second molars was planned, and the extracted teeth would be used to produce powder-type ATBGM for use at time of implant placement.

The mandibular left and right second molars were extracted and then used to produce powder-type ATBGM. Three months after the extractions, a mucoperiosteal flap was elevated on the right second molar site to attempt implant placement, but primary stability of the implant was impossible because the extraction socket had not healed sufficiently (Figs 13-5b and 13-5c). Powder-type ATBGM was placed in the socket (Fig 13-5d), which was then covered with a resorbable collagen membrane (BioGide) and sutured (Fig 13-5e). An implant (Superline, 4.8 mm in diameter, 6-mm platform, 8 mm in length) was placed 3 months after bone grafting with a primary stability of 71 ISQ (Figs 13-5f to 13-5h). Stage-two surgery was performed 2 months after implant placement, and the implant was at 85 ISQ (Figs 13-5i and 13-5j). The definitive prosthesis was performing properly 7 months after placement (Fig 13-5k).

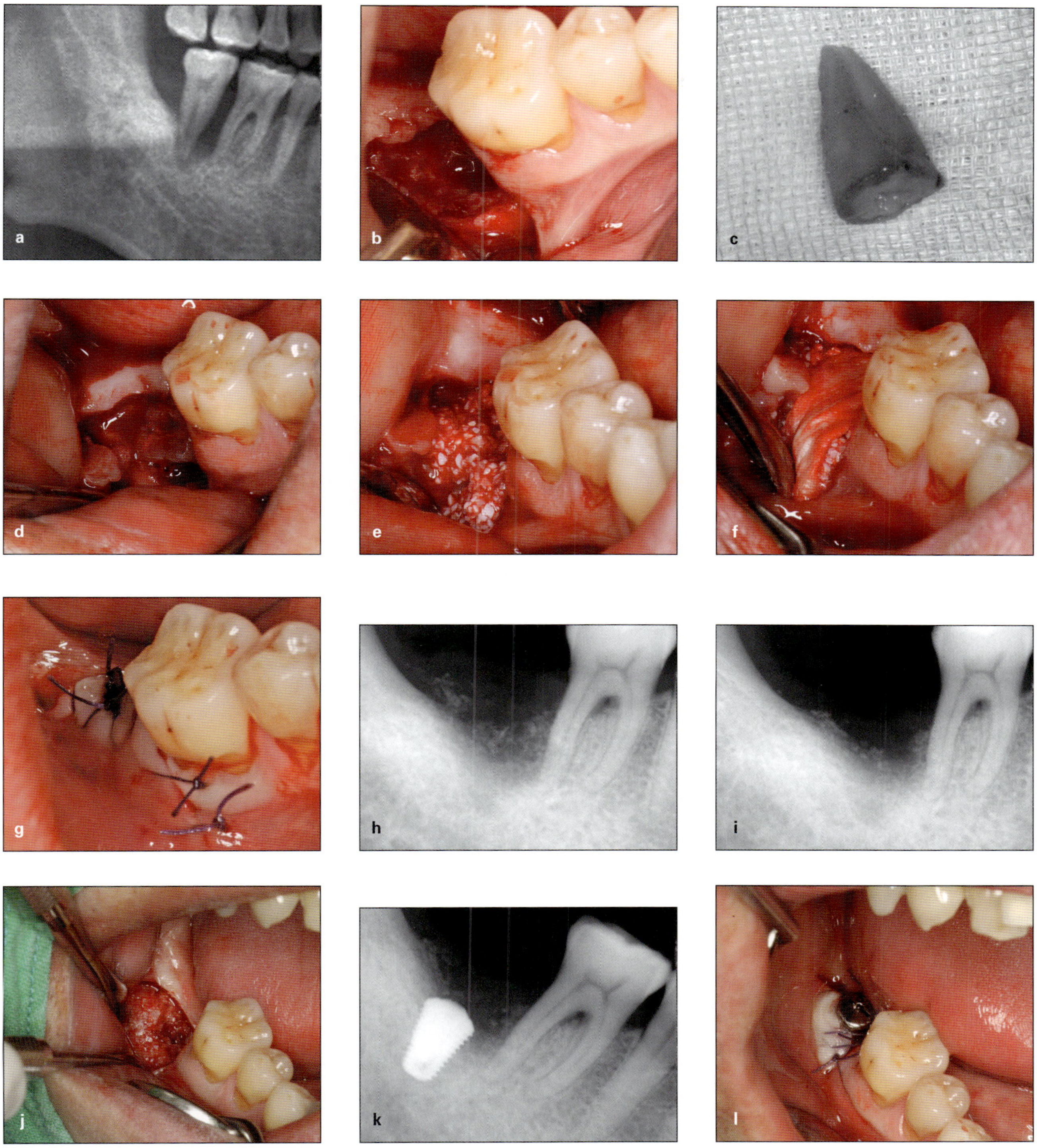

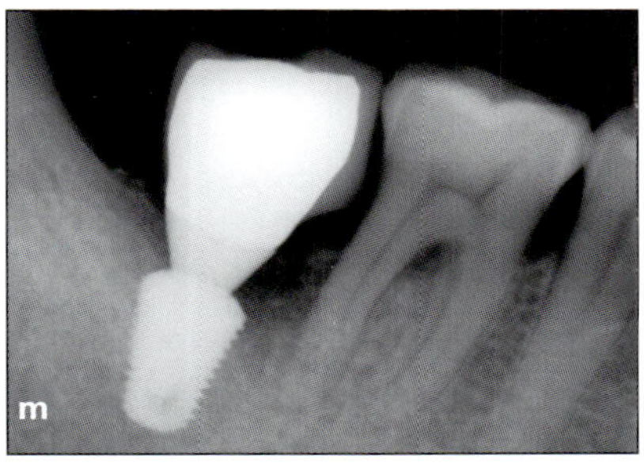

Fig 13-4 *(a)* At initial diagnosis. The mandibular right second molar needed to be extracted. *(b)* Elevation of a mucoperiosteal flap. *(c)* Block of ATBGM. *(d)* The ATBGM block in the extraction socket. *(e)* Powder-type ATBGM placed around the block. *(f)* The area was covered with a resorbable membrane. *(g)* The wound was sutured. *(h)* Periapical radiograph 1 week after bone grafting. *(i)* Periapical radiograph 5 months after bone grafting. *(j)* Elevation of a mucoperiosteal flap revealed that bone healing was very successful. *(k)* Periapical radiograph 1 week after implant placement. *(l)* Stage-two surgery. *(m)* Periapical radiograph 1 month after definitive prosthesis placement.

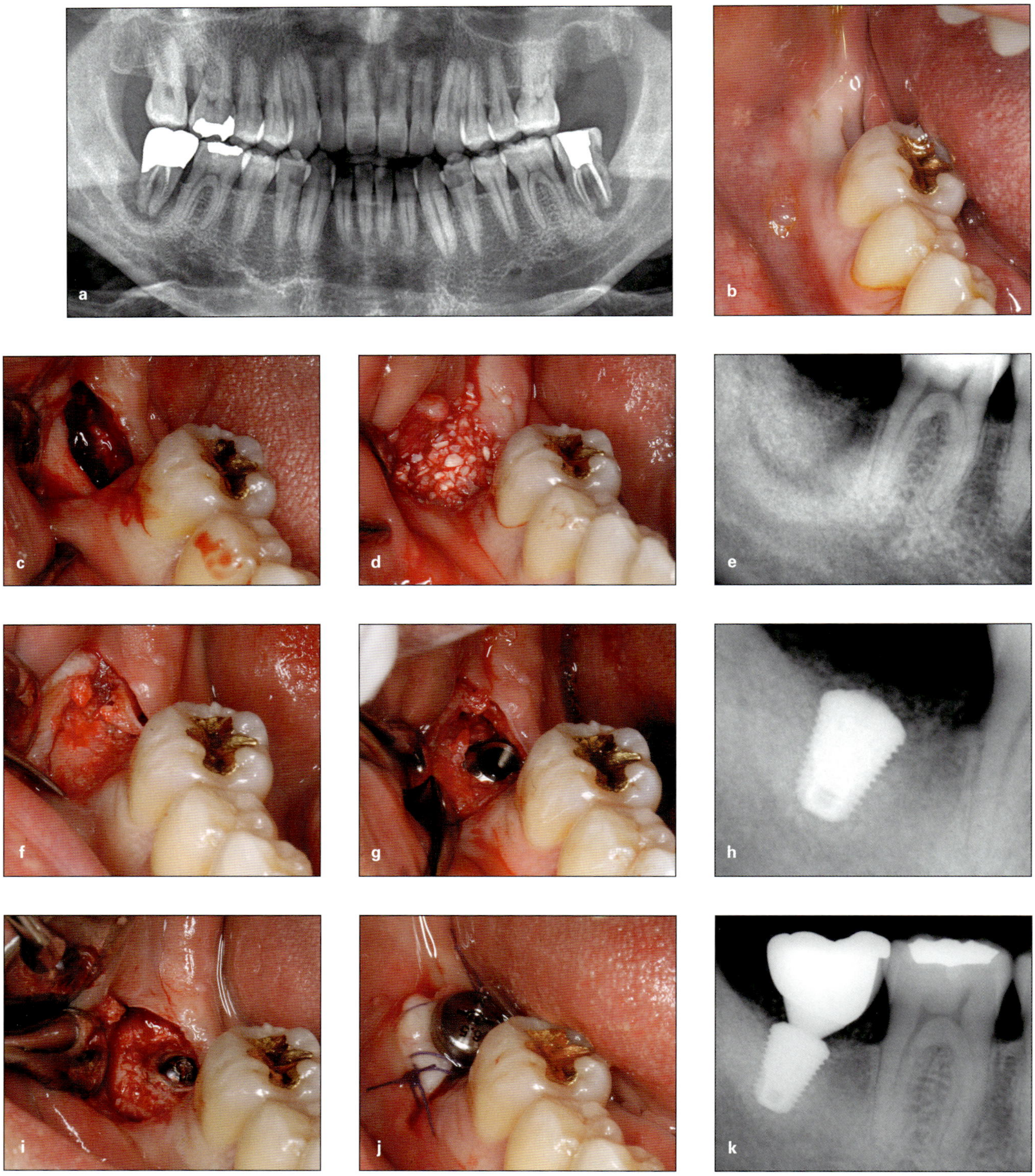

Fig 13-5 *(a)* At initial diagnosis. *(b)* At 3 months after extraction of the mandibular right second molar. *(c)* Elevation of a mucoperiosteal flap revealed that the extraction socket was almost completely unhealed; primary stability of an implant was not possible. *(d)* ATBGM in place. *(e)* After grafting of the extraction socket. *(f)* Elevation of a mucoperiosteal flap; bone healing was very successful. *(g)* Implant placement with good primary stability. *(h)* At 10 days after implant placement. *(i)* Implant exposed at stage-two surgery. *(j)* A healing abutment was connected, and the wound was sutured. *(k)* At 7 months after placement of the definitive prosthesis.

References

1. Tan WL, Wong TL, Wong MC, Lang NP. A systematic review of post-extractional alveolar hard and soft tissue dimensional changes in humans. Clin Oral Implants Res 2012;23(Suppl 5):1–21.
2. Darby I, Chen ST, Buser D. Ridge preservation techniques for implant therapy. Int J Oral Maxillofac Implants 2009;24(suppl):260–271.
3. Rothamel D, Schwarz F, Herten M, et al. Dimensional ridge alterations following socket preservation using a nanocrystalline hydroxyapatite paste: A histomorphometrical study in dogs. Int J Oral Maxillofac Surg 2008;37:741–747.
4. Becker W, Clokie C, Sennerby L, Urist MR, Becker BE. Histologic findings after implantation and evaluation of different grafting materials and titanium micro screws into extraction sockets: Case reports. J Periodontol 1998;69:414–421.
5. Shi B, Zhou Y, Wang YN, Cheng XR. Alveolar ridge preservation prior to implant placement with surgical-grade calcium sulfate and platelet-rich plasma: A pilot study in a canine model. Int J Oral Maxillofac Implants 2007;22:656–665.
6. Lekovic V, Camargo PM, Klokkevold PR, et al. Preservation of alveolar bone in extraction sockets using bioabsorbable membranes. J Periodontol 1998;69:1044–1049.
7. Neiva RF, Tsao YP, Eber R, Shotwell J, Billy E, Wang HL. Effects of a putty-form hydroxyapatite matrix combined with the synthetic cell-binding peptide P-15 on alveolar ridge preservation. J Periodontol 2008;79:291–299.
8. Luczyszyn SM, Papalexiou V, Novaes AB Jr, Grisi MF, Souza SL, Taba M Jr. Acellular dermal matrix and hydroxyapatite in prevention of ridge deformities after tooth extraction. Implant Dent 2005;14:176–184.
9. Iasella JM, Greenwell H, Miller RL, et al. Ridge preservation with freeze-dried bone allograft and a collagen membrane compared to extraction alone for implant site development: A clinical and histologic study in humans. J Periodontol 2003;74:990–999.
10. Sclar AG. Preserving alveolar ridge anatomy following tooth removal in conjunction with immediate implant placement. The Bio-Col technique. Atlas Oral Maxillofac Surg Clin North Am 1999;7:39–59.
11. Gross J. Ridge preservation using HTR synthetic bone following tooth extraction. Gen Dent 1995;43:364–367.
12. Camargo PM, Lekovic V, Carnio J, Kenney EB. Alveolar bone preservation following tooth extraction: A perspective of clinical trials utilizing osseous grafting and guided bone regeneration. Oral Maxillofac Surg Clin North Am 2004;16:9–18.
13. Serino G, Biancu S, Iezzi G, Piattelli A. Ridge preservation following tooth extraction using a polylactide and polyglycolide sponge as space filler: A clinical and histological study in humans. Clin Oral Implants Res 2003;14:651–658.
14. Kim YK, Kim SG, Byeon JH, et al. Development of a novel bone grafting material using autogenous teeth. Oral Surg Oral Med Oral Pathol Oral Radiol Endod 2010;109(4):496–503.
15. Artzi Z, Weinreb M, Tal H, et al. Experimental intrabony and periodontal defects treated with natural mineral combined with a synthetic cell-binding peptide in the canine: Morphometric evaluations. J Periodontol 2006;77:1658–1664.
16. Valentini P, Abensur D, Densari D, Graziani JN, Hämmerle C. Histological evaluation of Bio-Oss in a 2-stage sinus floor elevation and implantation procedure. A human case report. Clin Oral Implants Res 1998;9:59–64.
17. Hämmerle CH, Chiantella GC, Karring T, Lang NP. The effect of a deproteinized bovine bone mineral on bone regeneration around titanium dental implants. Clin Oral Implants Res 1998;9:151–162.

14

Periodontal and Peri-implant Defects

Kyung-Wook Kim, Bu-Kyu Lee

The major purpose of periodontal surgery is to provide an environment in which the periodontal tissues can be retained over the long term by removing and controlling plaque. Periodontal surgery is indicated when it is difficult to approach scaling or root planing as the result of *(1)* an increase in the depth of the periodontal pocket; *(2)* an increase in the width of teeth; or *(3)* incomplete coverage at the gingival crevice, a depression on a dental root, a bifurcation, or a subgingival portion of a tooth. Surgery is also indicated when an area becomes difficult for the patient to access for plaque control.

The various periodontal surgery techniques include gingivectomy, periodontal flaps, regeneration, molar surgery, alveoloplasty, and alveolar bone resection. Many different methods have been used for periodontal regeneration, and a variety of bone grafting materials have been used, including autogenous bone, allogeneic bone, xenogeneic bone, and alloplastic bone. Other approaches to periodontal regeneration include the use of citric acid or tetracycline for demineralization of dental roots and other methods that are believed to improve the biocompatibility of dental roots or promote cellular reactions. Physical barriers may be used to separate gingival connective tissues from a healing site and to keep the epithelium from approaching the dental root; this is the foundation of the concept of guided tissue regeneration.

Since implant dentistry became popular, the frequency of peri-implantitis has also increased. There is no single recommended treatment method for peri-implantitis. Roos-Jansåker et al[1] studied implants that were between 9 and 14 years old and reported that the depth of peri-implant pockets was greater than 4 mm on more than 48% of implants, and 7.7% of sites displayed bone loss. This emphasizes the importance of the prevention and treatment of peri-implantitis.

There are surgical and nonsurgical means to treat peri-implantitis according to the formation of the mucoperiosteal flap; nonsurgical methods can be clinically effective for a short period of time but generally do not provide positive long-term effects. Decontamination of implants can be achieved by mechanical or chemical measures.

Treatment of Peri-implantitis

Nonsurgical

Chemical treatment includes cleansing with chlorhexidine, local application of chemicals at the gingival crevice, or systemic antibiotic therapy. Occlusal treatment may be provided if there is early contact in occlusion or occlusal

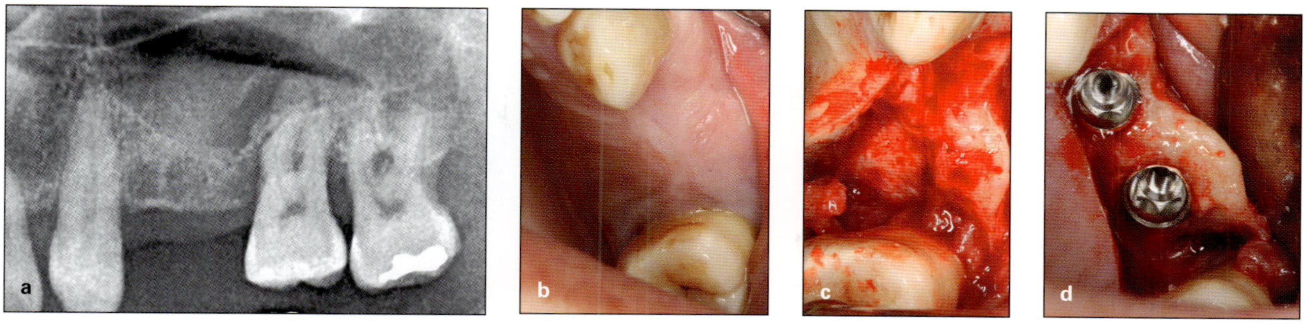

Fig 14-1 *(a)* Preoperative panoramic radiograph. *(b)* Preoperative intraoral view of the maxillary left quadrant. *(c)* Elevation of a mucoperiosteal flap revealing severe destruction of the alveolar bone around the maxillary first molar. *(d)* Implants placed in the premolar areas.

disharmony. Also, it can be helpful to wear protective appliances, since parafunctional habits (grinding or clenching) can overload the implants. Finally, mechanical treatment can be effective: A plastic or ultrasonic tool with a plastic tip may be used to remove inflammatory tissues, or a rubber cup with pumice or other air-powder abrasives can be employed to clean the implant surface.

Surgical

Surgery can be used to remove toxins from the surface of a contaminated implant. Regenerative or resective surgery may be performed, or the implant may be removed.

Literature review

Claffey et al[2] searched the literature published up to November 2007 on PubMed. Forty-three papers were reviewed.

- Animal studies revealed that: *(1)* reosseointegration can occur on a contaminated surface, *(2)* the condition of the surface plays a critical role in regeneration and reosseointegration, *(3)* no single particular method of surface decontamination is most effective, and *(4)* open debridement for decontamination can treat peri-implant lesions.
- Clinical studies led to the following conclusions: *(1)* there is no single particular method of surface decontamination that is most effective; and *(2)* the success rate of regeneration through bone grafting varied, regardless of the use of membranes; however, the purpose of regeneration is to fill in the bone defect, not to eliminate the lesion completely.

The clinical prognosis of bone grafting performed to regenerate periodontal bone defects or bone defects around implants is not certain. However, the survival of natural teeth and implants can be extended if defects are filled with bone graft materials and protected from inflammation over the long term. There is no definite information known about the ideal bone grafting materials, but the authors believe that the use of autogenous tooth bone graft material (ATBGM) can be safe for patients and as effective as autogenous bone grafting. Kim et al[3] confirmed that ATBGM underwent gradual resorption and was replaced by new bone of excellent quality through osteoinduction and osteoconduction.

Case Reports

Patient 1

A 56-year-old man sought treatment for missing maxillary left premolars and restoration of the mandibular right second molar (Figs 14-1a and 14-1b). He smoked more than 1 pack of cigarettes a day. Clinical examination revealed severe alveolar bone loss and a very poor periodontal condition. The seriously mobile maxillary right second molar and mandibular right second molar would be extracted and processed into powder-type ATBGM prior to planned implantation. The maxillary left first molar showed a grade III furcation involvement, but flap curettage with implantation was planned, as the patient wished to avoid extraction.

The maxillary right and mandibular right second molars were extracted and stored as powder-type ATBGM. A month later, a crestal incision was placed in the maxillary left premolar area and a gingival crevicular incision was placed above the maxillary left first molar to elevate a mucoperiosteal flap (Fig 14-1c). For the premolars, sinus elevation was performed through a crestal approach, and the enamel part (AutoBT enamel) of ATBGM was used. Implants were then placed (Osstem TS III SA; first premolar: 4 × 10 mm; second premolar: 4 × 8.5 mm) (Fig 14-1d).

When the inflammatory lesion around the maxillary left first molar was removed, bone loss to the tip of the palatal dental root with grade III furcation involvement could be seen. The root of this tooth was treated with tetracycline solution, and the wound was irrigated (Fig 14-1e). To treat the remaining bone defect around the first molar, the dentin portion (AutoBT dentin) of ATBGM was used, and the area was sutured (Figs 14-1f and 14-1g). In addition, an implant was placed in the mandibular left second molar area on the same day (Fig 14-1h).

At 3.5 months after surgery, stage-two surgery was performed for the implants in the maxillary left premolar area

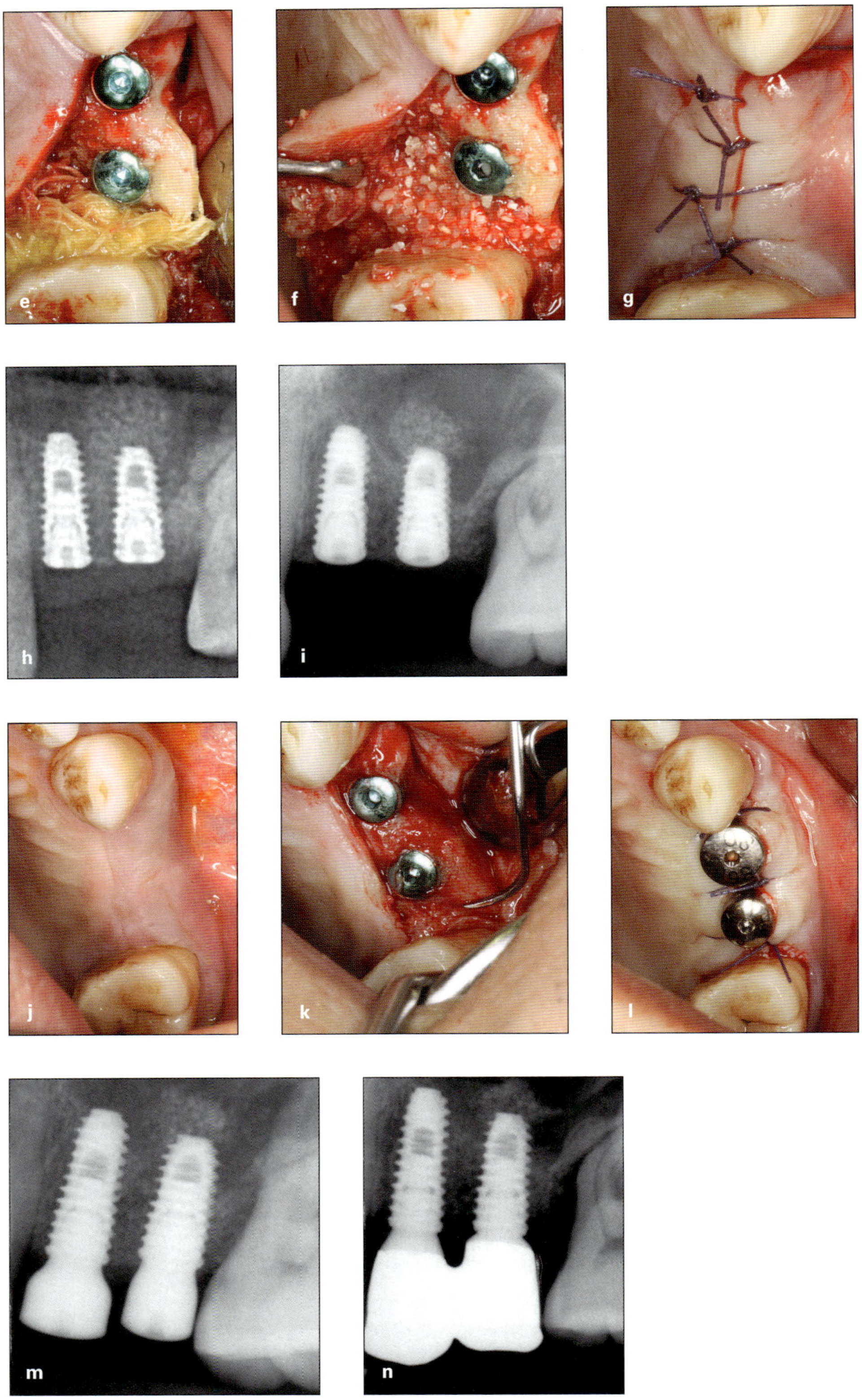

Fig 14-1 *(cont) (e)* Tetracycline was used to detoxify the dental root around the first molar. *(f)* Inflammatory tissues around the first molar were completely removed, and ATBGM was used to fill the defect. *(g)* The wound was sutured. *(h)* Postoperative panoramic view. *(i)* Periapical radiograph 3.5 months after surgery shows the ATBGM placed via sinus elevation at the apex of the second premolar implant. *(j)* Intraoral view prior to stage-two surgery. *(k)* Elevation of a mucoperiosteal flap revealed successful healing of the bone graft material in the mesial periodontal pocket of the first molar. *(l)* The healing abutments were connected. *(m)* Periapical radiograph after stage-two surgery. *(n)* Periapical radiograph 1 month after placement of the definitive prosthesis.

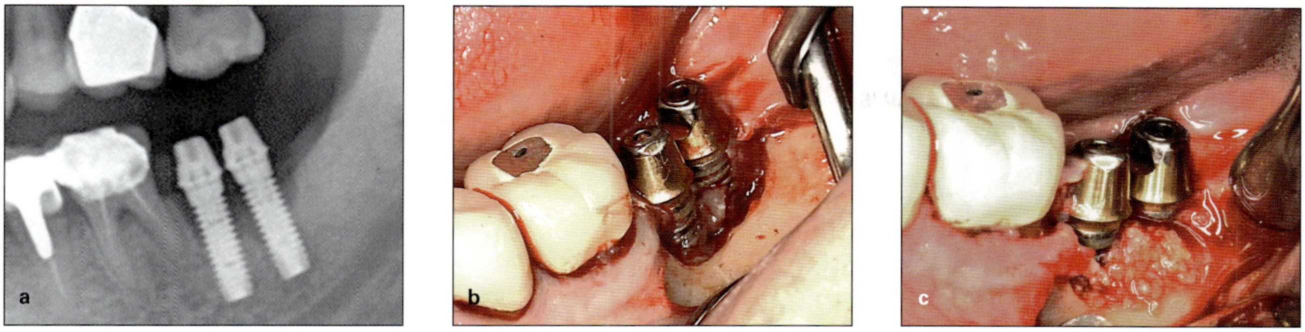

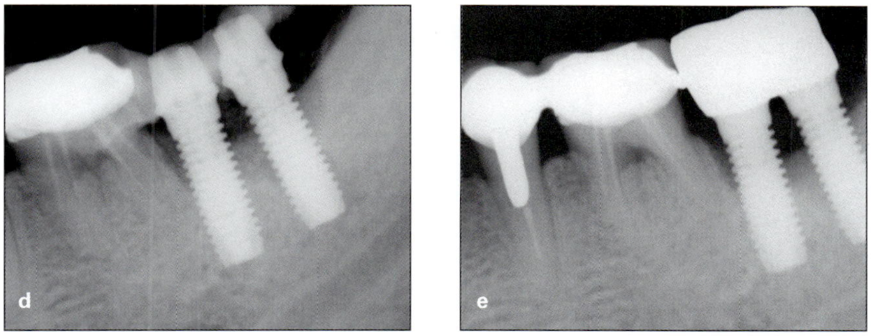

Fig 14-2 *(a)* Radiographic view at initial diagnosis. *(b)* Elevation of a mucoperiosteal flap revealed a serious bone defect. *(c)* The inflammatory tissues were removed, the surfaces of the implants were detoxified, and ATBGM was placed to fill the defects. *(d)* Postoperative periapical radiograph. *(e)* Periapical radiograph 10 months after surgery.

(Figs 14-1i and 14-1j). When a mucoperiosteal flap was elevated, it could be seen that the ATBGM around the first molar had healed successfully and the mobility was significantly reduced (Figs 14-1k to 14-1m). Two months following stage-two surgery, a definitive prosthesis was inserted (Fig 14-1n).

Patient 2

A 52-year-old man presented with gingival swelling and bleeding around implants in the mandibular left second and third molar areas that had been placed 5 years previously. Clinical and radiographic examinations showed deep periodontal pockets (second molar: buccal 6 mm, distal 9 mm, lingual 9 mm; third molar: buccal 7 mm, mesiodistal 9 mm, distal 6 mm, lingual 7 mm) and loss of alveolar bone, but the implants remained stable (Fig 14-2a). The hopeless mandibular right first and second molars were planned for extraction to produce ATBGM for treatment of the mandibular left molar implant sites.

The mandibular right first and second molars were extracted to produce ATBGM. One month later, a mucoperiosteal flap was elevated with local anesthesia to expose the mandibular left molar implants (Fig 14-2b). All inflammatory granulation tissues were removed, and tetracycline solution and an erbium:yttrium-aluminum-garnet laser were used to detoxify the implant surfaces. ATBGM was grafted into the defects, the wound was sutured, and healing abutments were inserted (Figs 14-2c and 14-2d). At a follow-up appointment 10 months later, the inflammation had disappeared around the implants, and the patient continued to receive regular maintenance treatment (Fig 14-2e).

Patient 3

A 74-year-old woman presented with a periapical abscess and periodontal abscess on the maxillary right second premolar and mesiodistal peri-implantitis on the maxillary right first molar implant. Radiographic examination showed increased radiolucency around the dental root of the maxillary right second premolar (Fig 14-3a). Extraction of the second premolar and replacement with an implant was planned, along with peri-implantitis treatment and bone grafting on the first molar implant.

Drainage was performed on the maxillary right second premolar, and antibiotic ointment was injected to treat buccal gingival swelling and pain. Two weeks later, flap curettage and laser treatment were performed on the maxillary right second premolar and first molar, but a foul odor and severe tenderness persisted when pressure was applied on the right side of the nose. Six months later, the second premolar was extracted and stored as powder-type ATBGM (Fig 14-3b). One month later, a mucoperiosteal flap was elevated over the area to expose the alveolar bone and the first molar implant (Fig 14-3c). The threads of the first molar implant were exposed. Ordinarily, the prosthesis connected to the adjoining implant (on the second molar) would be removed, but when this is clinically impossible or too difficult, surgery must be performed without removing the prosthesis. Inflammatory granulation tissues were removed around the exposed implant, which was then detoxified with tetracycline solution. An implant was placed in the second premolar area (Osstem GS III; 4 × 13 mm) (Fig 14-3d). ATBGM was placed in the surrounding bone defect and on the mesiodistal portion of the first molar implant (Fig 14-3e), collagen membrane

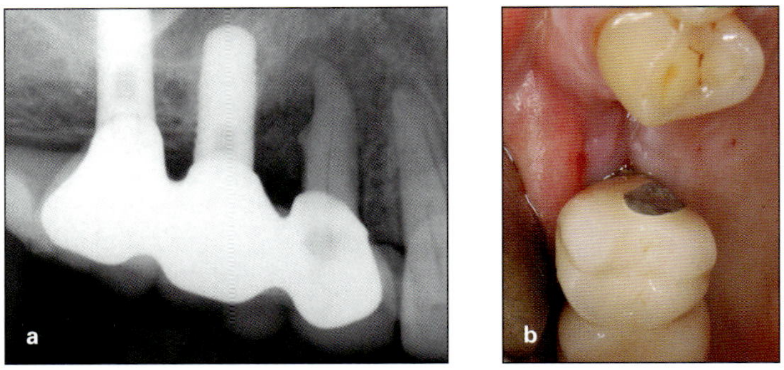

Fig 14-3 *(a)* Periapical radiograph at initial diagnosis. *(b)* Preoperative intraoral view 3 weeks after the extraction. *(c)* A mucoperiosteal flap was elevated above the second premolar and first molar. *(d)* An implant was placed in the second premolar area; a severe buccal dehiscence was observed. *(e)* ATBGM was placed around the implants and covered with Ossix Plus. *(f)* Periapical radiograph 10 days after implant placement and bone grafting. *(g)* The premolar area exposed for stage-two surgery. Successful bone healing was observed. *(h)* A healing abutment was connected, and the wound was sutured. *(i)* Periapical radiograph 9 months after definitive prosthetic treatment.

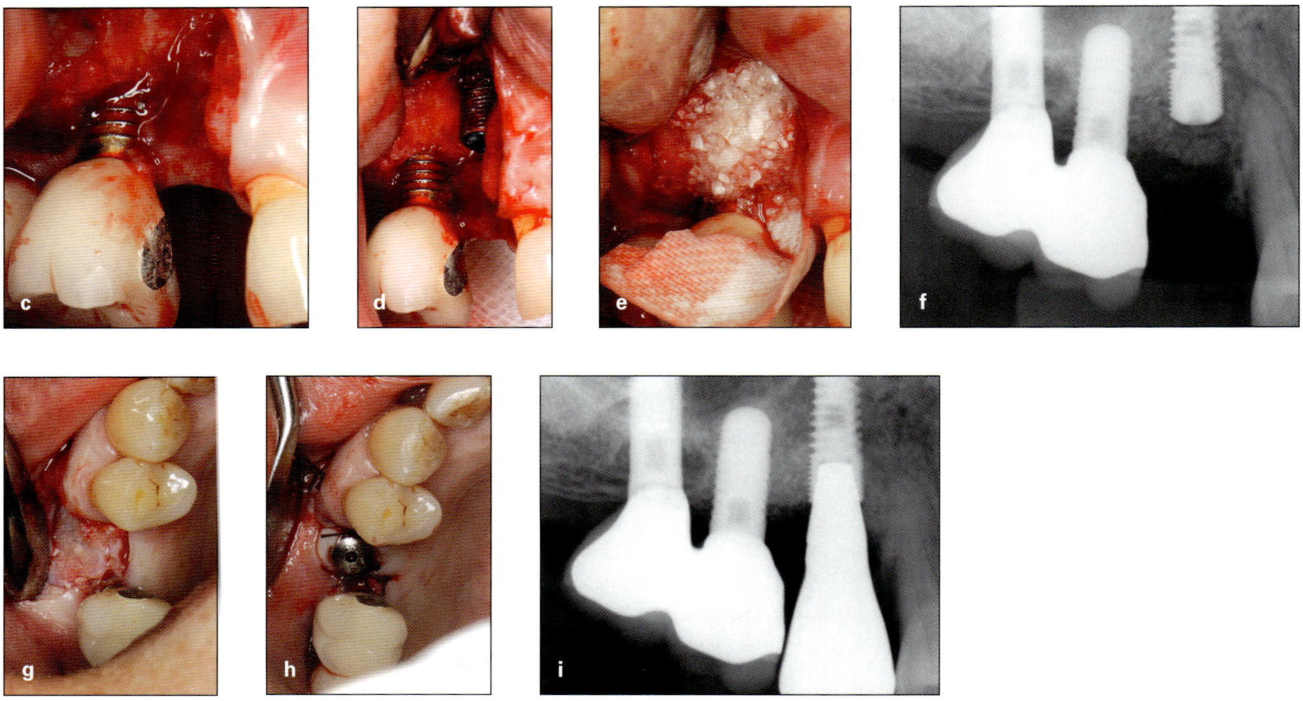

(Ossix Plus, Datum Dental) was used to cover the area, and wound closure was performed. The site was allowed to heal (Fig 14-3f). Stage-two surgery was performed 4 months later (Figs 14-3g and 14-3h). The definitive prosthesis was placed the following month and was working well 9 months later (Fig 14-3i).

References

1. Roos-Jansåker AM, Renvert H, Lindahl C, Renvert S. Nine- to fourteen-year follow-up of implant treatment. Part III: Factors associated with peri-implant lesions. J Clin Periodontol 2006; 33:296–301.
2. Claffey N, Clarke E, Polyzois I, Renvert S. Surgical treatment of peri-implantitis. J Clin Periodontol 2008;35(8 suppl):316–332.
3. Kim YK, Kim SG, Byeon JH, et al. Development of a novel bone grafting material using autogenous teeth. Oral Surg Oral Med Oral Pathol Oral Radiol Endod 2010;109:496–503.

15

Familial Tooth Bone Graft

In-Woong Um, Jeong-Keun Lee

It has been reported that allogeneic tooth bone graft between parents and their offspring or between siblings may delay or reduce immunologic reactions if the tissue-located histocompatibility antigens (H-antigens) are compatible. Kim et al[1] anticipated good results when a tooth from a 9- to 11-year-old child, scheduled for removal in conjunction with orthodontic treatment, is grafted to treat a tooth defect in his or her parent or sibling.

An extracted tooth can be processed and stored to produce bone graft material in a manner similar to that normally used to produce autogenous tooth bone graft material, and it may then be used by other directly related family members (siblings, parents, or offspring) for treatment. The kinds of teeth that can be extracted and donated include any teeth that cannot be preserved through dental surgery, primary teeth, and third molars. Dental offices must obtain a donor agreement and a beneficiary agreement as well as an agreement to process the extracted tooth when a tooth is extracted for donation to a family member. After the donor and beneficiary agreements are prepared, they are signed by the donor (or the parents, when necessary). The donor is examined for hepatitis, sexually transmitted diseases, and HIV, but examinations may be added or omitted when requested and agreed upon by the donor and the beneficiary. The beneficiary must provide confirmation of the familial relationship with the donor and must sign the beneficiary agreement.

The term *isograft* refers to a graft between genetically identical entities (eg, monozygotic twins). Because monozygotic twins will have an identical major histocompatibility complex, there is no chance of graft rejection. Therefore, this is the most preferred type of graft in organ transplantation. An isograft is generally classified as an autogenous graft. Tooth bone grafting between direct family members involves almost no risk of immune rejection, as the donors and recipients have a similar genetic complex and the graft material is processed through demineralization and freeze-drying. Demineralized allogeneic bone graft materials do not require histocompatibility testing, such as ABO typing. Because grafting materials obtained from family members are processed through demineralization, special histocompatibility testing is not necessary.

Barrett and Reade[2–4] performed tooth isografting in mouse renal subcapsular sites and assessed the result histologically. They observed the formation of alveolar bone and periodontal ligaments on teeth with incomplete roots. They reported that teeth with complete dental roots did not form alveolar bone or periodontal ligaments. In that study, alveolar bone formed after isografting of incomplete teeth because of osteoconduction and an indirect osteoinductive mechanism. An experimental study published in 1982 of a premature molar isograft of a mouse in intraosseous and extraosseous sites observed that bone formation occurred in the kidney and the tibia.[5]

Steidler and Reade[6] studied the effect of length of time of a graft outside the body with teeth isografting in rodents. They observed changes in size, necrosis of cementum, resorption of the dental root, and osseointegration when the teeth remained outside the body for more than 30 minutes. The study also observed new bone forma-

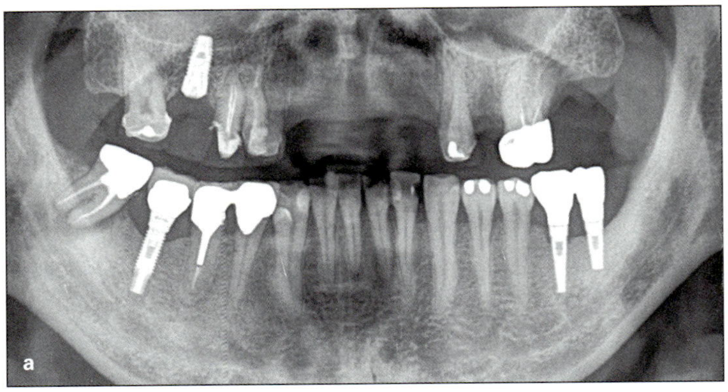

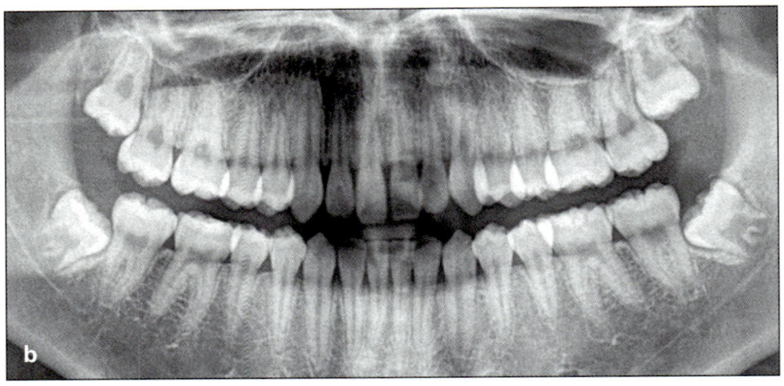

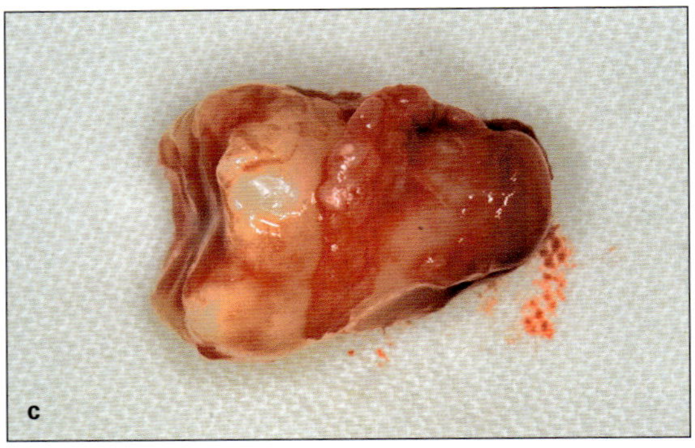

Fig 15-1 *(a)* Panoramic view at initial diagnosis. The patient was referred for horizontal augmentation of the alveolar bone. *(b)* Panoramic view of the patient's 15-year-old daughter showing impacted maxillary and mandibular third molars. *(c)* An impacted third molar extracted from the 15-year-old adolescent girl.

tion around tooth isografts in the tibia, which was assumed to be a result of osteoinduction by the teeth.

Barrett et al[7] conducted an immunologic study of tooth isograft in mice. They performed isografts of the third mandibular molars of mature mice into tibial shaft medulla and renal subcapsular kidney sites. Six months later, they performed histologic testing to observe the initial changes at both sites and observed constant regeneration with formation of dentin. The tibial shaft isograft was surrounded by bone, and constant resorption from the coronal dentin was observed. The teeth grafted at the subcapsular kidney site were not surrounded by bone and showed no resorption of the crown. Teeth isografts on intraosseous parts displayed various degrees of root resorption and osseointegration. However, reformation of the periodontal ligament was not observed. They observed decreases in the number and array of mature periodontal ligament fiber bundles, production of fibers parallel to the dental root, and decreases in the thickness of surrounding alveolar bone. The authors stated that such degenerative changes of periodontal ligament tissue were likely a result of the nonfunctional state of the isografted teeth. They continued: "We observed constant regeneration of new tubular dentine in an experimental study on isograft of incomplete teeth with remaining periodontal ligament. Also, we observed bone formation in both the kidney and the tibia. Despite the formation of dentin and cementum, however, there was no formation of normal dental root because there was no epithelial root sheath."[7]

The following case reports illustrate the use of familial tooth bone graft material in different clinical situations.

Patient 1

A 45-year-old man was referred for ridge augmentation in the anterior maxilla (Fig 15-1a). The dentist had planned to place implants in the areas of both maxillary canines to support a six-unit fixed prosthesis, but the diameter of the buccolingual ridge was too narrow. The authors therefore planned to extract a third molar from the patient and two impacted third molars from his daughter to produce tooth bone graft material in both block and powder forms for bone grafting.

The patient's mandibular right third molar was extracted and processed into powder-type bone graft material. On the same day, impacted third molars were extracted from his daughter (Figs 15-1b and 15-1c) and stored as block-type and powder-type bone graft material (Fig 15-1d). Two weeks later, block-type bone graft was hydrated in saline solution for 30 minutes and divided in half with a no. 15 blade (Fig 15-1e). Skin flaps were elevated over the anterior maxilla beginning with a crestal incision, and the block-type bone

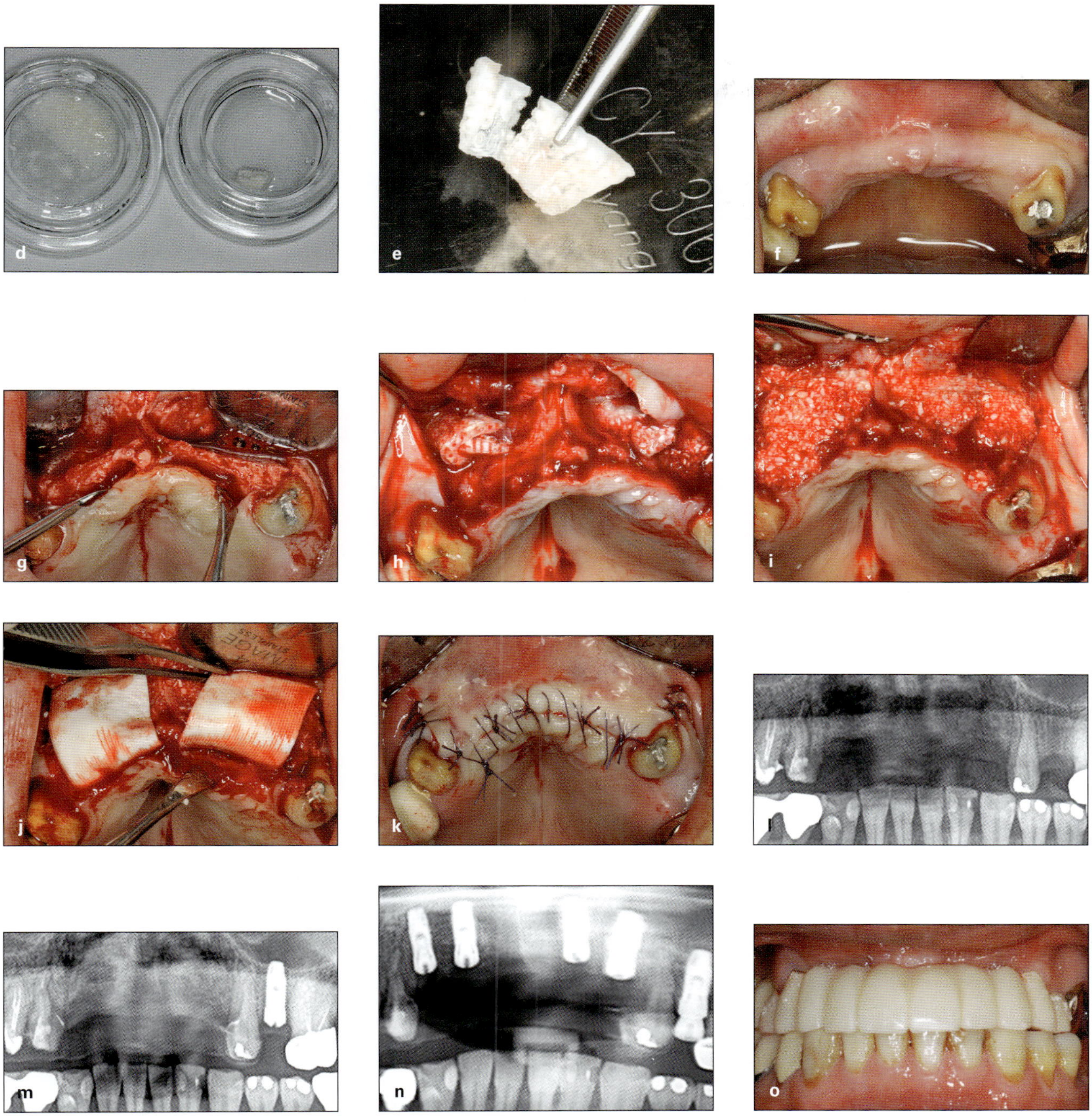

Fig 15-1 *(cont) (d)* The daughter's impacted tooth was processed into powder-type *(left)* and block-type *(right)* bone graft material. *(e)* The hydrated block-type bone graft material was divided in half and spread. *(f)* Preoperative intraoral view. *(g)* Elevation of a mucoperiosteal flap revealed the narrow buccolingual ridge. *(h)* The blocks were placed; no screws were used for fixation. *(i)* Powder-type bone graft material in place. *(j)* The site was covered with a collagen membrane. *(k)* The site was sutured. *(l)* Postoperative panoramic view. *(m)* At 3.5 months after bone grafting. *(n)* Panoramic view after implant placement. *(o)* Provisional implant-supported prosthesis in place.

grafting material was placed on the labial side of both canine sites, with powder-type bone graft material added around it (Figs 15-1f to 15-1i). The areas were covered with a resorbable collagen membrane (Ossix Plus, Datum Dental), and the wound was sutured (Figs 15-1j to 15-1l). Bone healing was successful and uncomplicated (Fig 15-1m). Four months later, the patient returned to his regular dentist for implant placement and restoration (Figs 15-1n and 15-1o).

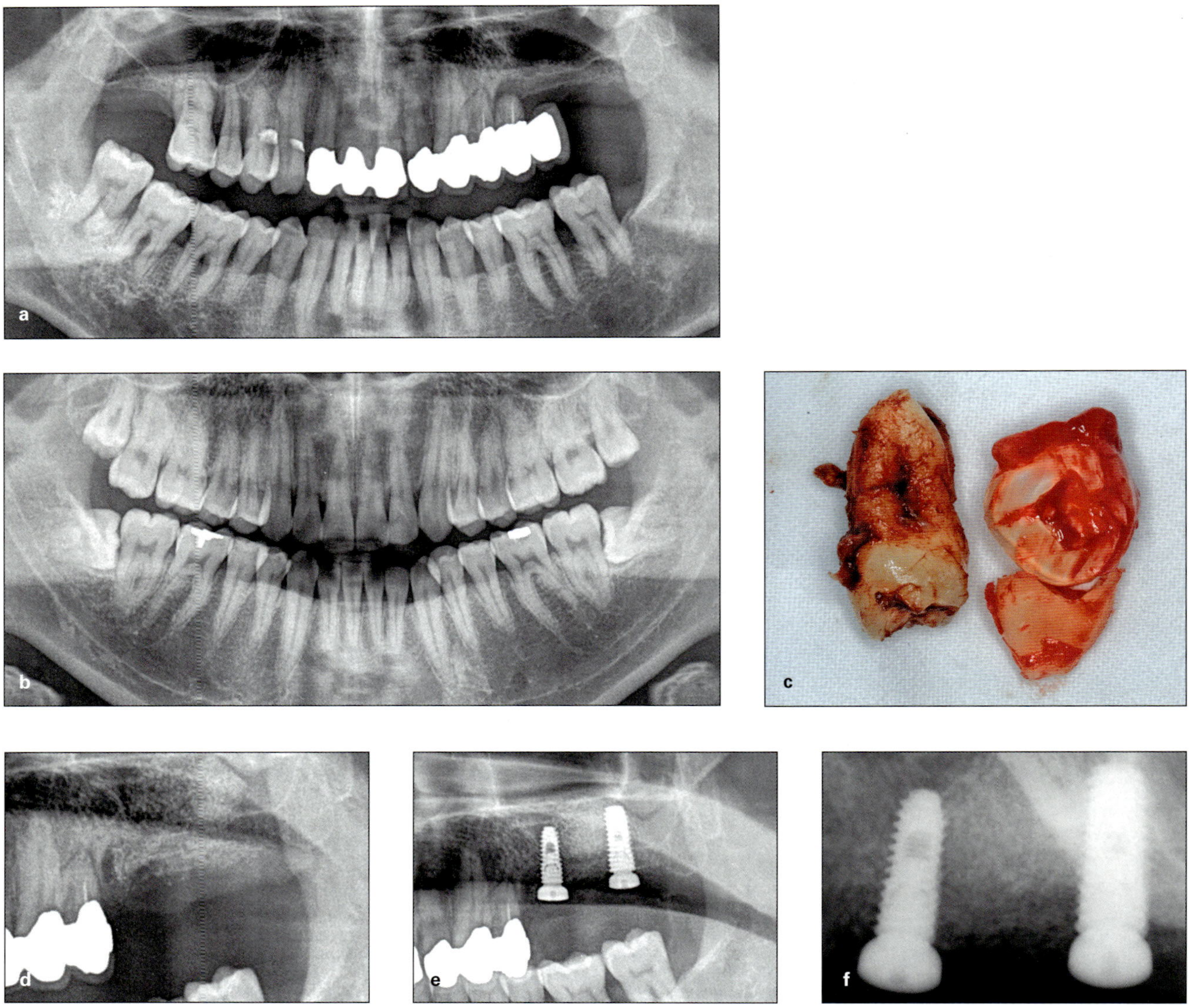

Fig 15-2 *(a)* Panoramic view at initial diagnosis. *(b)* Panoramic view of the patient's 22-year-old son. *(c)* Third molars from the patient's son. *(d)* Panoramic view after sinus elevation. *(e)* Panoramic view after implants were placed (3 months after bone grafting). *(f)* Periapical radiograph after implant placement

Patient 2

A 49-year-old man presented with pain in the maxillary left second premolar area and wanted implants in the neighboring first and second molar areas (Fig 15-2a). A periapical abscess at the premolar was diagnosed, and extraction of the tooth was planned. The patient's impacted mandibular right third molar and his son's impacted third molars would be used to produce bone graft material for a planned sinus elevation in the posterior left maxilla, followed by delayed implant placement.

The patient's mandibular right third molar was extracted, and the maxillary right and mandibular third molars from the patient's 22-year-old son were extracted to produce powder-type bone graft material (Figs 15-2b and 15-2c). Two weeks later, the prosthesis was cut between the maxillary left premolars, and the second premolar was extracted. A crestal incision was made from the second premolar to the second molar, and a mucoperiosteal flap was elevated to perform sinus elevation through a lateral approach. The autogenous tooth graft material and powder-type tooth graft material from the son were used (Fig 15-2d). Implants (Osstem TS III; 4.0 × 11.5 mm at the second premolar, 5.0 × 11.5 mm at the second molar) were placed 3 months later using a single-stage method, and the implant stability quotients (measured by Osstell Mentor) were 67 at the second premolar and 71 at the second molar. A healing abutment was connected, and the wound was sutured (Figs 15-2e and 15-2f). The definitive prosthesis was delivered 5 months after implant placement.

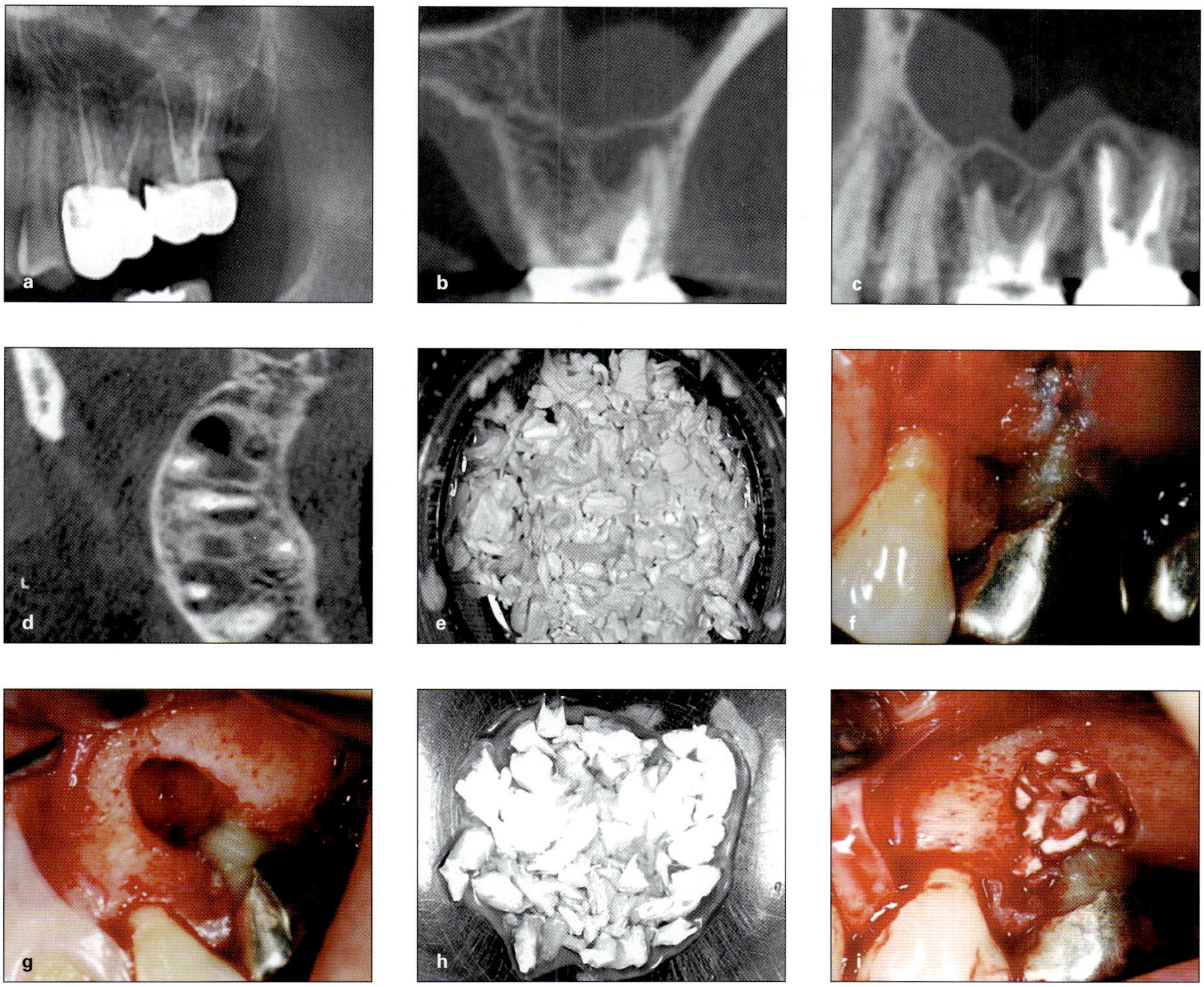

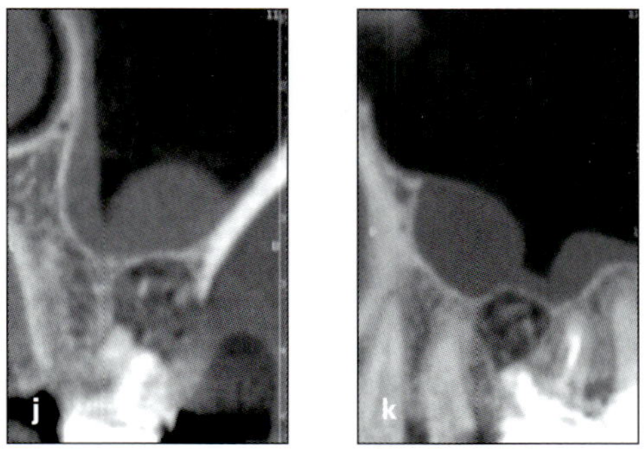

Fig 15-3 *(a)* Panoramic view at initial diagnosis. *(b to d)* CT images at initial diagnosis. *(e)* Chip-type bone graft material created from the son's third molar. *(f)* Elevation of a mucoperiosteal flap exposed the cyst. *(g)* The cyst was removed. *(h)* The familial tooth bone graft chips. *(i)* Chips after placement in the defect. *(j and k)* Postoperative CT views.

Patient 3

A 52-year-old woman presented with pain in the area of the maxillary left first molar. Radiographs and computed tomographic (CT) scans revealed a severe bone defect and an enucleated cyst on the buccal dental root of the maxillary left first molar (Figs 15-3a to 15-3d). The sinus membrane showed thickening. The patient requested bone grafting with a tooth from her son after cyst enucleation.

The son's third molar was extracted to produce chip-type tooth bone graft material (Fig 15-3e). A mucoperiosteal flap was elevated to expose the cyst for removal (Figs 15-3f and 15-3g). The familial tooth bone graft chips were hydrated in saline solution prior to grafting and then placed in the bone defect (Figs 15-3h and 15-3i). The patient's pain was relieved, and bone healing was successful (Figs 15-3j and 15-3k).

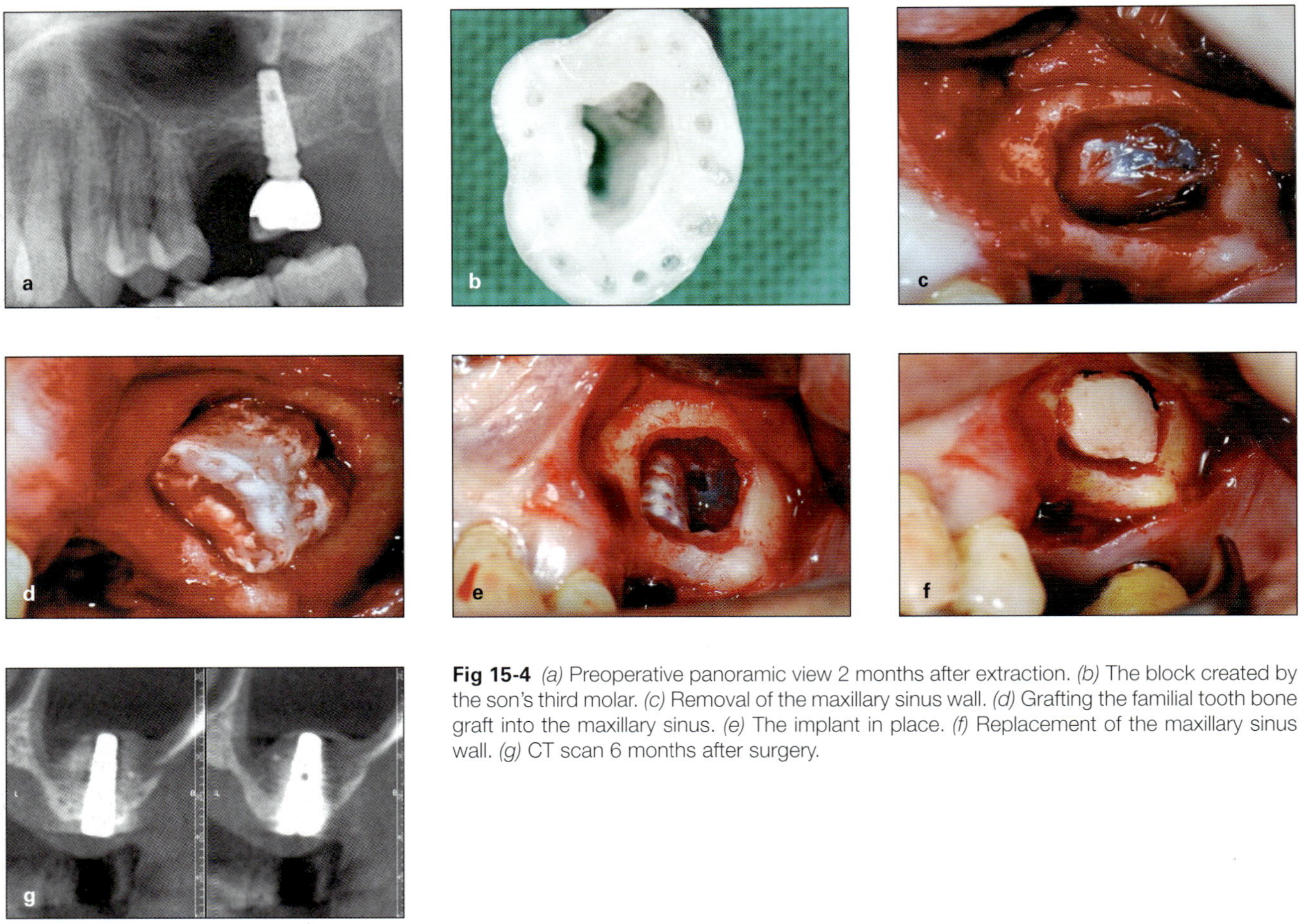

Fig 15-4 *(a)* Preoperative panoramic view 2 months after extraction. *(b)* The block created by the son's third molar. *(c)* Removal of the maxillary sinus wall. *(d)* Grafting the familial tooth bone graft into the maxillary sinus. *(e)* The implant in place. *(f)* Replacement of the maxillary sinus wall. *(g)* CT scan 6 months after surgery.

Patient 4

A 51-year-old man presented with pain in the maxillary left first molar area. Clinical and radiographic examination revealed a cyst, and the decision was made to extract the tooth and place an implant.

The height of the alveolar bone apical to the maxillary sinus was too low, so sinus bone grafting through a lateral approach was required (Fig 15-4a). Familial tooth material was created using his son's extracted third molar. Because of the size and dimensions of the maxillary sinus area, the authors opted to use block-type tooth graft material (Fig 15-4b). Two months after extraction of the tooth, the patient's sinus membrane was elevated using a lateral approach. The maxillary sinus wall was removed to visualize the maxillary sinus membrane (Fig 15-4c). The block-type familial tooth bone graft was placed into the maxillary sinus followed by simultaneous implant placement (Figs 15-4d to 15-4f). The graft was successful (Figs 15-4e to 15-4g).

References

1. Kim SJ, Kim YM, Kim MR. Present and future of the autogenous tooth graft. Dent Clin 2010;30:790–800.
2. Barrett AP, Reade PC. Changes in periodontal fibre organization in mature bone/tooth isografts in mice. J Oral Pathol 1981;10:276–283.
3. Barrett AP, Reade PC. A histological investigation of isografts of mature mouse molars to an intrabony and an extrabony site. Transplantation 1981;31:353–357.
4. Barrett AP, Reade PC. The relationship between degree of development of tooth isografts and the subsequent formation of bone and periodontal ligament. J Periodontal Res 1981;16:456–465.
5. Barrett AP, Reade PC. A histological investigations of isografts of immature mouse molars to an intrabony and extrabony site. Arch Oral Biol 1982;27:59–63.
6. Steidler NE, Reade PC. An histological study of the effects of extra-corporeal time on murine dental isografts. Arch Oral Biol 1979;24:165–169.
7. Barrett AP, Reade PC. Revascularization of mouse tooth isografts and allografts using autoradiography and carbon-perfusion. Arch Oral Biol 1981;26:541–545.